HARLAXTON COLLEGE

R218

D1586405

LI c c/ WIL

NA
HEALERS

UNIVERSITY OF EVANSVILLE
HARLAXTON COLLEGE LIBRARY
HARLAXTON MANOR
GRANTHAM, LINCS

NATURAL BORN
HEALERS

HOW TO FIND THE BEST
COMPLEMENTARY HEALTH TREATMENTS
FOR YOU AND YOUR FAMILY

**ELISABETH WILSON &
DR GEORGE LEWITH** MRCP MRCGP

UNIVERSITY OF EVANSVILLE
HARLAXTON COLLEGE LIBRARY
HARLAXTON MANOR
GRANTHAM, LINCS

A CHANNEL FOUR BOOK

First published in Great Britain in 1997
by Collins & Brown Limited
London House
Great Eastern Wharf
Parkgate Road
London SW11 4NQ

Published in association with Channel Four Television Corporation and based on the series
produced for Channel Four Television by Wild and Fresh Productions.

Copyright © Collins & Brown Limited 1997

Text copyright © Elisabeth Wilson & George Lewith 1997

The right of Elisabeth Wilson & George Lewith to be identified as the author of this work has
been asserted by them in accordance with the Copyright, Designs and Patents Act, 1988.

All rights reserved. No part of this publication may be reproduced, stored in a retrieval system,
or transmitted in any form or by any means, electronic, mechanical, photocopying, recording or
otherwise, without the prior written permission of the copyright owner.

1 3 5 7 9 8 6 4 2

British Library Cataloguing-in-Publication Data:
A catalogue record for this book
is available from the British Library.

ISBN 1 85585 446 5

Editor: Mary Lambert
Designer: Paul Wood

Printed and bound in Finland by WSOY

about the authors

Dr George Lewith MA DM MRCP MRCGP is a complementary medical physician, acupuncturist and homoeopath and an academic, and is co-director of The Centre for the Study of Complementary Medicine in Southampton. He is also an Honorary Senior Lecturer in the Department of Medicine at Southampton University and he acted as a consultant on the Channel 4 series 'Natural Born Healers'.

Elisabeth Wilson has a degree in medical science and has worked as a health journalist for over 10 years. She is currently Health Editor on *SHE* magazine and has written for many newspapers and magazines.

ACKNOWLEDGEMENTS

A big thank you to all the people I interviewed in the course of researching this book who very generously gave me their time. Special thanks to Charlotte Black, for her invaluable interest and support, and to Izzie Pick, for allowing me to draw on her excellent research. Thanks also to acupuncturist Lynn Osborne for her input and without whose help this book wouldn't have got written – EW.

This book is not intended as an alternative to personal medical advice. The reader should consult a doctor in all matters relating to health and particularly in respect of any symptoms which may require diagnosis or medical attention. The authors cannot take responsibility for the treatment recommendations of individual therapists.

contents

foreword

My interest in complementary medicine began in the late 1970s when I went on an acupuncture course to China and realized that as a highly trained conventional doctor there were treatments out there which could significantly benefit patients and with which I had had virtually no contact. I then began to learn about how to apply a variety of these techniques clinically, in particular acupuncture, manipulative therapies, environmental medicine, nutritional medicine and homoeopathy. As my clinical interest and expertise developed, I became progressively fascinated by a large number of unanswered questions that related to these various complementary medical approaches, specifically how they work and in what situations they should be best used.

It seems that more and more people wish to have treatment through a variety of 'natural' or complementary medical approaches. We have tried as far as possible to evaluate the research available on a broad range of conditions so that we can offer help and advice to those in need. Many of the therapies we discuss have not been extensively evaluated, but a lack of research certainly does not mean that the therapy is ineffective, simply that it has not been adequately researched.

The advice given in this book is the culmination of 20 years of clinical work and research within the broad area of alternative medicine. I hope this advice will benefit those who want to explore this area as a means of improving their health.

Dr George Lewith, University of Southampton School of Medicine.

introduction

When I was suffering from a particularly painful and unattractive form of eczema, complementary medicine came to my rescue when orthodox medicine had failed. I am a convert. I can say – melodramatically but all the same truthfully – that complementary medicine has changed my life. It cured me, and it also intrigued me. Since then I have tried various different therapies and all of them have helped me to become a healthier and less stressed person.

But complementary medicine also frustrates me. It was only a stroke of luck that I found the right form of treatment at the very time when I needed help most. I doubt others are so fortunate. As a journalist, whose job primarily is to supply useful information, I find the whole area distressingly woolly. I field calls from people on a daily basis who although open to complementary medicine don't know where to begin. Would their arthritic hip benefit more from acupuncture or nutritional medicine? Does homoeopathy cure asthma? Is there any evidence that a particular herbal supplement will alleviate their depression? They know that complementary medicine works – they just don't know which therapy will work for them.

This book is an attempt to deliver some reassurance. We have taken a number of illnesses and conditions and then, based mainly upon the scientific evidence so far, recommended which one or two, of the eight main therapies, you can feel confident is most likely to help with your particular ailment. This does not mean that other therapies have nothing to offer but complementary treatment can be costly; we've taken this route because as a potential patient, it can be comforting to know that you are opting for a treatment that has been shown to help others before you.

There is a lot to criticize in this approach. Complementary medicine is not an exact science. Unlike orthodox medicine, it works on many, very subtle levels, and the most obvious one is the enormous benefit to the patient of a good patient-therapist relationship. If there's a cure this rapport is usually there, but you can't measure it.

The nub of the problem with taking the scientific approach in evaluating complementary therapies is that patients often feel 'better' almost instantly for having had the therapy, but their symptoms may still be present for some time. Knowing this, complementary therapists are often loath to have their therapies put through scientific models of evaluation. They have ample evidence that their treatments work, and long waiting lists to prove that the public thinks so, too. Although there is a growing band who are prepared to submit their therapies for research, most (although not all) don't see the necessity of proving anything or of undertaking their own research to the level that would be accepted by sceptical medics. However, an increasing band of doctors around the world who recognize the worth of complementary medicine have started to put it under the scientific microscope, and it is their research which is the basis of this book.

In short, scientific research can't tell the whole story about complementary medicine but it can form the framework of a starting-off point for the consumer who wants to know 'which therapy for me?'

We can perhaps look forward to a day when there will be a perfectly integrated system of treatment to help patients get the very best from orthodox and complementary medicine together. The Research Council for Complementary Medicine is already working on such a model for asthma, but admits that coming up with a cogent method of dealing with just one disease involving both orthodox and complementary medicine is fraught with problems. In the meantime, everyone has to rely, as we have here, on a mixture of scientific research and anecdotal reports of healing in making a decision about which therapy to go for.

Why try complementary medicine?

If you are thinking about trying a complementary therapy, it's probably for one of the following reasons.

● Orthodox medicine has failed you.

● You are receiving orthodox treatment, or contemplating it, but do not want to take drugs long-term to manage your symptoms – you want a cure.

● You want to take more control of your own health – the natural way.

Despite the difficulties of knowing which therapy to try, and whether it works, the interest in complementary medicine is growing. In 1993, it was Europe's second biggest growth industry after microelectronics. In 1995, according to a Consumers' Association survey in Great Britain, one in four people had tried it in the previous 12 months (an almost 100 per cent increase in six years; back in 1989, it was one in seven). About two-thirds of those seeking it were women, but both men and women report equal satisfaction with their treatment although men are more likely to look for a quick solution to an immediate health problem, whereas women are more likely to undergo treatment as part of a search for a more healthy lifestyle.

Orthodox medicine works for the most part on one level – it works as a 'fix-it' for a particular symptom or illness. Complementary medicine can often act as a 'fix-it', too. If that's what you want, this book can tell you which treatments should work fastest for your particular problem.

However, many patients seeking out complementary medicine want more. They may start off with an immediate problem which needs treatment, but they are also aware that their general health isn't good. (This is borne out by the fact that nothing appears to be physically wrong with 40 per cent of patients who visit their doctors.)

All of us love the idea of being treated holistically, and nod enthusiastically when told by the therapist that he or she will be treating our mind, body and spirit as one, without having a clue, really, of what that entails (certainly that was my own experience). In practice, it often means that as our body heals, our mind and spirit are given the space to heal, too. We start with one therapy, take what we need from it and then deciding to take the healing process another stage, move onto another, usually with the blessing of our original therapist. Our body energy shifts little by little until we heal ourselves. With complementary medicine, we start to listen to our bodies and take control of our own health, and that can be an exhilarating experience.

From the patient case histories in this book you will see that many have tried several therapies in their search for wellbeing and although this book aims to give you one or two ideas to start off with, be aware that these one or two have a good chance of helping but they may not be the whole solution. Your instincts, and your therapist's knowledge, will be the best guide to what you might need next.

How effective is complementary medicine?

There have been many trials to assess how pleased patients are with complementary medicine. An overview of 14 of these concluded 'that a considerable proportion . . . perceived it as effective'. A *Which? Health* survey of 1995 found that overall three-quarters of the patients who had tried complementary medicine felt that their condition had improved as a direct result, and 83 per cent felt that their general sense of wellbeing had improved. (Of the therapies covered in this book, osteopathy, chiropractic, acupuncture and healing all had over 80 per cent satisfaction levels. Herbalism and homoeopathy were in the high 70s. Hypnotherapy had around 50 per cent satisfaction. Nutritional medicine and clinical ecology weren't surveyed.)

It is thought by many experts that as complementary medicine becomes more mainstream, the number of reports of patient dissatisfaction will grow – purely because more patients will be trying the therapies. But it is hoped that if more conclusive research is forthcoming, along the lines of the pioneering work Dr George Lewith and his colleagues are carrying out in researching and integrating therapies with orthodox medicine, patients will feel better informed before they embark on treatment, and so avoid any potential pitfalls.

If you are looking for a cure, I hope the information in this book goes some way in helping you achieve it.

Elisabeth Wilson

Complementary medicine is so diverse that it is difficult to find a single theme or philosophy that unites all the different therapies. It is probably fair to say that the approaches within complementary medicine aim to enhance the body's response to illness and to allow for a natural healing process as opposed to conventional medicine, which in many chronic conditions simply aims to suppress symptoms. The complementary medical approach to illness, particularly chronic illness, therefore allows the body to work at its best so we can heal ourselves. How do the therapies achieve this?

● Nutritional medicine, clinical ecology, herbalism and homoeopathy help to strengthen the body's immune system and biochemical functioning so that the body as a whole 'works' much better.

● Acupuncture and healing strengthen the body's immune, hormonal and endocrine systems, freeing up the flow of energy and removing any blockages.

● Mind–body therapies relax the mind and focus it. This leads to definite beneficial physiological effects.

● Osteopathy and chiropractic make structural changes in the body which allow better functioning of the immune, hormonal and endocrine systems.

A major stumbling block for many sceptical Westerners is the way that ancient therapies discuss this energy. For instance, when a therapist talks of 'poor liver energy' when there is nothing obviously wrong with the liver, it is easy to dismiss the whole therapy. But this method of talking about energy is only a 'model' – a framework on which to base treatment. A Traditional Chinese Medical (TCM) practitioner can talk about someone having 'good liver energy' even when that patient's liver has been removed. It is simply a shorthand for the type of person they are dealing with just as Western doctors will talk of a Type A person to signify a patient who is driven, stressed out, a perfectionist and likely to die of a heart condition if they don't slow down. These ancient models of disease work when used by well-trained therapists within the context of their therapeutic disciplines.

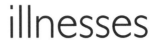

illnesses

For details of all the therapies mentioned below,
see Chapter 3, pages 83–140.

ANXIETY

It would be an unusual person who didn't feel anxious at some point in their daily lives. But anxiety attacks in response to stress, fear and in some cases for no apparent reason are a different matter and can be severely debilitating to the patient. Orthodox medicine treats anxiety by teaching breathing techniques to cope with 'panic' attacks or with drugs – sedatives or tranquillizers (which can be addictive if taken for too long). Since attacks are usually accompanied by an increased heart rate, beta-blockers which affect the heart rate are also sometimes given.

Complementary medicine can work very well for some anxious patients, and gives them back a sense of control over what can be a frightening group of symptoms. It does this without any of the side effects of conventional drug treatment.

Where to start?

There may be no easy cure. Mind–body therapies such as yoga and meditation have an instant calming effect and in the long-term, can cure anxiety. (Hypnotherapy is also particularly useful if the anxiety takes the form of a phobia.) If the anxiety is due to nutritional deficiency, the improvement following appropriate supplementation, under the guidance of a nutritional therapist, can be dramatic. Changing your diet might make a difference as there is definite evidence that certain foods cause anxiety (see box on page 17). However, eliminating foods from your diet may take several months to show a clear improvement.

Once nutritional considerations are taken out of the equation, homoeopathy and healing are also worth considering as treatments.

NUTRITIONAL MEDICINE

Anxious people have been shown to be deficient in certain key nutrients, and taking supplements can help them.

● Vitamin B appears to be particularly important. Twelve patients suffering from agoraphobia were found to be deficient in several of the B group vitamins. When 23 patients (including these 12) were given dietary advice, multivitamins and large doses of the vitamins in which they were found to be deficient, 19 had a dramatic improvement three months later (11 of these 19 became free of panic attacks) (1).

● Serotonin is a chemical which transmits messages at nerve endings and a deficiency of it can lead to anxiety. Another natural chemical, tryptophan, is needed to produce serotonin and depressed patients have often been found to be low in it. When patients prone to hyperventilating were given tryptophan along with pyrodoxine (one of the B vitamins), 70–80 per cent showed improvement (2).

FOODS TO AVOID IF PRONE TO ANXIETY

● **Caffeine**
● **Sugar and sugary foods**
● **Tea**
● **Chocolate**
● **Alcohol**

All these foods and drinks have been shown to make anxiety states worse. Avoiding them for three to four months can help, but you have to be strict about it, as 'relapses' can bring on quite dramatic symptoms. It is best to avoid these foods completely to maintain any benefit, but usually after about four months you become sensitized to them and can tolerate small amounts, about twice a week, at the very most. A clinical ecologist or nutritional therapist can help to give you further advice.

HOMOEOPATHY

There are no clinical trials that have tested homoeopathy for anxiety but many people find it useful. 'Classical' homoeopathy, where the patient profile matches the remedy will have the best results, but the following remedies may give some clue as to the variety of anxiety states which can be helped.

Symptom	Remedy
For people whose apprehension leads to diarrhoea.	Argentum nitricum
For individuals who are constantly restless, pace up and down a lot and are often overly tidy.	Arsenicum album
For people who wake up nervous, wanting fresh air, and who have a tendency to faint.	Carbo veg
For people who cannot act as they are paralysed by anxiety and fear.	Gelsemium

HEALING

There are widespread reports of how well anxious patients respond to 'therapeutic touch' and in the United States it is used to calm patients in hospital.

One way of experiencing therapeutic touch is through massage and this can be useful in anxiety. However, it is not the massage per se but the therapeutic touch element which is essential and so, not just any old massage is of use. In other words, it is not the movement of the hands which matters, but the concentration of the therapist. A well-trained aromatherapist is ideal. Any good one will give the necessary 'focused attention' to the patient which is necessary for healing. (Anxious patients given a back rub with therapeutic touch showed improvement; without the therapeutic touch, the massage didn't do so much good [3]).

THERAPEUTIC TOUCH

Therapeutic touch is similar, if not for all practical purposes, identical, to healing. The difference is one of emphasis. Here, in Great Britain, although there is a surprising acceptance of healing by the medical profession, it is still seen in rather mystical terms – healers are 'born' with their gift and normally discover for themselves that they have it.

In the United States where therapeutic touch is much more commonly offered to patients, especially by nurses, it is seen as a technique that can be taught, although the therapist has to be a compassionate person, able to focus completely on the patient, without becoming overly involved or hung up on proving that she can heal them.

The assumption is made that energy fields are the fundamental units of all living things and that humans are whole beings and should never be seen purely in terms of their parts. The aim is to rebalance the energy field of the patient, relaxing them (possibly through massage) and so facilitating the healing process.

During therapeutic touch, the therapist becomes centred and focused on the patient. The practitioner's hands are placed close to, or gently laid on, the patient's body and slowly moved over the body to assess subtle changes in the body's energy. She is looking for blocked or low-energy areas. Then the therapist focuses her attention on specific areas of the body in order to rebalance and redirect the patient's energy.

It is particularly useful for pain relief and anxiety but see pages 120–124 for more details of where healing is appropriate (or inappropriate).

ARTHRITIS

The definition of arthritis is 'inflammation of the joints'. There are two kinds: osteoarthritis and rheumatoid arthritis. If you suffer from either condition conventional drugs can help, but there is no cure for either type of arthritis short of surgery although this can often greatly help patients. However, the painful acute attacks can be minimized and daily life made more bearable with careful management, and that is what complementary medicine can offer the patient.

Osteoarthritis

Where two bones meet, a joint is formed. Cushioning each bone surface are two layers of cartilage, surrounded by a capsule of fluid (synovial fluid) which together protect the bone and allow smooth movement. As we grow older, natural wear and tear means the cartilage thins causing osteorarthritis.

It has been suggested that by the age of 60, most people will have some sign of this disease, although we will not all develop symptoms. Being overweight plus the cumulative effects of a lifetime of inadequate exercise and diet can contribute towards osteoarthritis developing. Hormonal fluctuations can also precipitate osteoarthritis; it can start during pregnancy and after the menopause. The joints affected are the ones that are used most, such as the ankles, knees, hips, spine and hands.

The symptoms of osteoarthritis include the following.

● Pain and stiffness, which is caused by the bones rubbing against each other without any protection. In an attempt to heal the affected joint, little spurs of bone grow into the joint and these also cause pain. It can be a disabling disease. Range of movement at the joint is decreased and it can be very difficult to 'get going' especially in the morning because of stiffness. However, often the disease does not seriously impair the function of the joints.

● Swelling, heat and redness which are due to inflammation at the joint. This is especially marked during acute attacks.

Osteoarthritis is usually treated with a group of drugs known as non-steroidal anti-inflammatory (NSAIDs), but these can have side effects such as stomach problems.

Although these drugs are useful, the side effects can make them unpalatable to patients. And it is often in order to cut down their drug consumption that patients start to look into alternative treatments in the first place.

Steroid injections are also given and treatment with water and heat can give some relief of symptoms. Anti-inflammatory gels can also be rubbed into the affected areas.

Where to start?

Specific studies into osteoarthritis are not plentiful, but acupuncture can help reduce the pain and inflammation and is worth trying. Herbal medicine has also been successful in decreasing the symptoms.

Food sensitivity may play a part in widespread osteoarthritis (but not if it is just present in one joint), Since NSAIDs have been shown to increase the permeability of the gut wall, and this may exacerbate symptoms of food sensitivity, patients who have widespread osteoarthritis should have this checked out by a clinical ecologist or nutritional therapist.

Homoeopathy and nutritional medicine may be helpful in treating osteoarthritis depending on the individual case.

ACUPUNCTURE

Osteoarthritis is a chronic (long-term), painful condition and acupuncture is a very effective method of treating the pain and can also bring long-lasting benefits. Forty patients were divided into two groups, one group receiving acupuncture at points known to relieve arthritic pain, the other at placebo points. Both groups reported having less pain and tenderness (1). In another study, this time of 25 patients with osteoarthritis in their cervical bones (in the neck), 75 per cent of the group receiving acupuncture as opposed to 31 per cent of the group receiving placebo reported less pain (2).

When the benefits of acupuncture against physiotherapy were looked at in osteoarthritis of the knee, there were significantly better results with acupuncture (3).

For the story of a patient treated with acupuncture for osteoarthritis, see pages 91–92.

HERBAL MEDICINE

An extract from the New Zealand green-lipped mussel has had good results in several tests to treat osteoarthritis due to its anti-inflammatory effects. *Hypericum perforatum* (St John's Wort) is also a potent anti-inflammatory, which in tests on rats gave comparable results to steroids (4).

HOMOEOPATHY

The treatments used in this therapy have been found to help relieve many of the symptoms of osteoarthritis, but the trouble with actually evaluating how much use homoeopathy is in treating osteoarthritis is that the studies carried out so far tend to pitch one drug against one homoeopathic treatment. But of course, for results with homoeopathy it is essential to match the treatment to the patient, so allowing just one homoeopathic prescription is not really giving 'homoeopathy' a fair chance.

However, homoeopaths often treat osteoarthritis patients. Even if the clinical evidence isn't there, it would appear to offer some relief. The following are among some of the treatments which can be used, depending on the patient profile.

For an acute attack the following may be prescribed.

Symptom	Remedy
For where there is a lot of swelling and redness.	Apis
For when the condition is worse for cold and damp.	Dulcemara
For pains which go from joint to joint.	Pulsatilla

For day-to-day chronic discomfort the following remedies may give some relief.

Symptom	Remedy
For when the patient is anxious and tends to move too fast causing accidents.	Argentum nitricum
For when gout is also present.	Cholchicum
For when there is muscle spasm.	Nux vomica
For when there is muscle stiffness protecting the affected joints, better after moving about a little.	Rhus tox
For when osteoarthritis starts in the menopause.	Sepia

NUTRITIONAL MEDICINE

Many sufferers from osteoarthritis have nutritional deficiencies or food allergies and their symptoms often improve once these are treated. A group of 29 patients took both 600mg vitamin E (in its natural form, tocopherol, which acts as an anti-inflammatory) and a placebo daily for 10 days each. Fifty-two per cent of the patients had less pain as opposed to 4 per cent while taking the placebo (5).

In another trial 35 per cent of patients taking green-lipped mussel in the dose of 1200 to 3000 mg for between six months to four years gained relief from their symptoms (6).

In a further study of patients suffering from arthritis (59 per cent had osteoarthritis) 61 per cent taking yucca saponin extract saw improvement in swelling, pain and stiffness as opposed to 22 per cent who were on placebo treatment. In some cases, there was improvement in a few days, although in other cases it took three months or longer (7).

Rheumatoid arthritis

This is an extremely painful condition where the joints become inflamed and painful. The patient also feels low, unwell and may lose weight. Exactly why it occurs isn't known, but it is thought that there may be an auto-immune connection, where the body's defence systems turn on itself, and this accounts for the painful inflammation. This inflammation can eventually cause the destruction of the joints so keeping the disease at bay is a major aim of both conventional and complementary treatment.

Aspirin is often prescribed and NSAIDs to relieve pain and stiffness. Other conventional drugs used to treat rheumatoid arthritis are powerful and can have negative side effects and this makes complementary medicine even more attractive to patients.

However, there is no complementary medicine that can compete with the relief which patients derive from joint replacement, which can sometimes prove necessary if the joint is damaged too badly.

Where to start?

For pain relief, acupuncture can work quickly. To alleviate the joint inflammation, it is worth looking at making changes in diet. Homoeopathy has also had good results in controlling inflammation.

There is also evidence that herbal medicine, clinical ecology and nutritional medicine can also help relieve the symptoms of rheumatoid arthritis.

ACUPUNCTURE

Acupuncture is effective in controlling about 70 per cent of chronic (long-term) painful conditions including rheumatoid arthritis. An overview of all the studies carried out on the effect of acupuncture on rheumatoid arthritis shows that it is successful (1). One study showed that acupuncture was more effective at treating knee problems than local steroid injections (2).

Relief can be obtained from 'needling' the points adjoining the afflicted joint. You can expect improvement within three to four sessions. If there is no improvement then acupuncture may not have anything to offer. How long the effect lasts is very variable, and of course badly damaged joints will probably need repeat treatments sooner. Relief can last for about three to six months, but the effect can last for as long as 18 months.

This pain relief applies when just the joint area is treated, which is the approach most likely to be taken by doctors offering acupuncture to patients. However, a traditional Chinese acupuncturist, although also able to offer quick pain relief, would as is common practice, expect to work for longer on a patient, dealing with healing the system as a whole. The aim of treatment would be to stimulate the immune system to deal with the rheumatoid arthritis and this can work well, although it takes much longer. However, the claims that acupuncture can treat inflammation are not backed up by clinical research while there is indisputable proof that it can help people to cope with the pain.

HOMOEOPATHY

Various remedies from this therapy have been found to help sufferers of rheumatoid arthritis. In connection with clinical trials, there was a surprisingly good result in one trial involving testing just one homoeopathic remedy, Rhus tox, against a placebo. This result was surprising in that only one treatment was used for all of the patients in the trial: usually for homoeopathy to work the remedy has to be tailored specifically for the individual patient. Nevertheless, Rhus tox gave the patients relief from their symptoms for at least a year after the treatment (3).

Treatment takes about two months, and it may take some time to find the right remedy for the patient which may prolong treatment for even longer. But if after nine months there is no improvement, it is unlikely that homoeopathy is the answer.

HERBAL MEDICINE

Green-lipped mussel has been found to be helpful for arthritic conditions, but it is particularly effective for rheumatoid arthritis. Of 60 patients who took the extract and the placebo (at different times!), 28 had rheumatoid arthritis and of these, 68 per cent reported an improvement with green lipped mussel as opposed to 35 per cent with placebo (4).

CLINICAL ECOLOGY

Arthritis Care report that 32 per cent of their members have tried to treat their arthritis by changing their diet. There are many different recommendations, but no hard and fast evidence that avoiding any one kind of food will reap positive benefits. Avoiding milk, wheat or meat (patients on vegetarian diets did better in one study [5]) is a good start.

However, arthritis may be triggered by almost any combination of foods. The only way to be sure that the right foods are being eliminated is to follow a very restricted diet and introduce foods gradually in order to determine triggers. It may take 24 hours for the return of symptoms after eating the trigger food, and several days for the pain to die down. This should always be done under the supervision of an expert, because there can be a real possibility of nutrient deficiency.

Once the trigger foods are identified and eliminated, you can expect to feel some improvement after six weeks. You will begin to feel substantially better after two to three months. This obviously takes a fair amount of discipline on the part of the patient, but the odd slip up isn't the end of the world as after a while the patient will probably become food tolerant (see pages 124–130).

NUTRITIONAL MEDICINE

Taking vitamin and mineral supplements has been found to reduce pain. Vitamin C may be useful because it fights inflammation and it has been suggested as particularly useful in rheumatoid arthritis (6). In a study of children with arthritis it was found that they tended to be deficient in both vitamin C and selenium and the conclusion was that supplementation would be useful (7).

Therapists are particularly fond of supplementing with zinc in cases of inflammation because it is so vital to the immune system, and it is easy for people to become depleted in zinc. Patients with psoriatic arthritis (another chronic disease of the joints) have benefited from zinc treatment (8) and it may have the same results in rheumatoid arthritis.

ASTHMA

Asthma is a debilitating disease of the respiratory system which makes breathing normally difficult. In serious attacks it can sometimes kill. For acute attacks, complementary medication has nothing to offer over conventional medication and the latter should always be used. There are two main types of conventional treatment: bronchodilators which increase air flow and immunosuppressives (oral or inhaled steroids) which 'damp down' the allergic response.

Asthma is on the increase, or at least the number of people who are receiving asthmatic medication is on the increase. Many sufferers (or parents of young sufferers) are loath to use powerful drugs to treat the ailment any more than is strictly necessary.

The drugs that are prescribed are aimed at suppressing the attack and do nothing to deal with the underlying cause of the asthma, the frequency of the attacks, or their severity when it strikes. It is here that complementary medicine can really help.

There are many causes of asthma and working out what is triggering the attacks in any one patient is often a complicated process. It can be hereditary and allergies to dust and dust mites, pollens and moulds, and environmental pollution have all been implicated. Emotional stress and even vigorous exercise can bring on attacks. Often more than one trigger is involved.

Where to start?

The good news is that there is a great deal that can be done by the patient. Asthma is a frightening condition and the psychological boost for asthmatics in feeling that they are to some extent in control of their own symptoms is an added bonus. There is clear evidence that the mind–body therapies can help, and this can give sufferers the desired feeling of having some control. They should be considered by all adult sufferers. Nutritional medicine and homoeopathy also have something to offer, especially when they are undertaken in conjunction with yoga or hypnotherapy.

Acupuncture, clinical ecology and herbalism also appear to have a positive benefit for some people, but more research is needed.

MIND–BODY THERAPIES

These therapies have been show to help asthma sufferers as they learn to gain some control over their bodies.

● **Yoga** has been shown to help asthma as reported in the British Medical Journal (1). Patients were asked to undertake an hour of special breathing and yoga positions, plus slow breathing and meditational exercises for six weeks. At the end of this time, the yoga patients were shown to have significantly less asthma symptoms, less attacks, and also decreased dependence on drugs than the patients who had equally severe symptoms at the beginning of the trial but who were not undertaking yoga.

● **Hypnotherapy** can improve symptoms and decrease the use of drugs after six weeks if you are in the 80 per cent of the population who are susceptible to hypnosis (2).

NUTRITIONAL MEDICINE

Vitamin and mineral supplements have been found to help reduce asthma attacks. In fact, available evidence suggests that asthma can be helped by supplementation with vitamin B6, vitamin B12, niacin, vitamin C and magnesium (3). Nutritional therapists also often suggest asthmatics avoid caffeine and there is evidence that sodium intake could be linked to asthma so avoiding sodium (found in salt and salty foods) may also help (4).

However, patients should always be assessed by a nutritional therapist to determine if vitamin/mineral supplementation or food elimination would actually benefit them; self-medication is unlikely to be helpful.

If progress is going to be made, you can expect it to happen within three to four months. However, where emotional stress acts as a trigger, mind–body techniques will be needed, too.

CLINICAL ECOLOGY

Food sensitivity can be a very important cause of asthma but is often overlooked because the symptoms appear hours, even days after the food has been eaten (5). If your asthma is linked to other allergic type symptoms such as eczema or a family history of an allergy, then it's worth considering that food allergy could be playing a part.

One particularly dramatic study illustrates this. It was carried out on 263 patients who were using steroids or bronchodilators. Avoiding certain foods resulted in steroid use dropping from 26 to 3 per cent, and bronchodilator use dropping from 44 per cent to 20 per cent (6).

The most common foods that asthmatic patients are allergic to are: milk, eggs, artificial colorants and wheat (more common in older than young patients).

HOMOEOPATHY

Where there is a definite link to be made between the onset of an asthma attack and an allergen, then homoeopathy could be the answer. The success depends on identifying the type of allergen correctly. A minute dose of the allergen can then prove beneficial (7). For instance, if asthma wheezing only happens in the summer when you are exposed to pollen, then a treatment with a homoeopathic preparation of pollen may help. Patients report that with homoeopathy their asthma symptoms were much improved and they were able to halve their use of the antihistamines used to treat hay fever (8).

Better controlled studies are needed but there is evidence that homeopathy can be useful in cases where specific triggers like house dust mites, moulds and pollen can be isolated.

BACK PAIN

You will have read many times that backache is part and parcel of being human – the ultimate price that we pay for walking upright. Certainly the statistics substantiate this: according to one study 60 per cent of individuals will complain of backache in any two-week period.

Back pain, however, is not something we have to endure. It is most often due to bad lifestyle choices. It is one condition that by taking preventative measures you can protect your spine from. Research, mainly carried out in the United States, has shown that much back pain is due to poor posture, being overweight and the 'couch potato' lifestyle. These all put cumulative strain on the spine until a minuscule movement triggers an excruciating attack. A common scenario is the lower back pain sufferer who spends most of his working day hunched in front of a computer screen and who has steadily put on weight since his teens. One day, he casually reaches for a coffee cup and experiences a sharp pain that shoots down his back incapacitating him for the next two weeks. This man may well take to his bed and treat himself with painkillers, the very action which will give him least benefit according to the latest thinking.

The traditional Western approach to back pain is geared towards alleviating the discomfort until the spine 'heals' itself and has little to offer cases of chronic (long-term) back pain, especially when it is occupational in origin. This is where complementary therapy has a lot to offer. In fact doctors have increasingly turned to these methods in an effort to offer their patients the very best care.

Where to start?

Whether your back pain is recent (acute) or long-term (chronic), there are two clear winners when it comes to treating lower back pain: the manipulative therapies – osteopathy and chiropractic – and acupuncture. Experience at The Centre for the Study of Complementary Therapy, Southampton, shows that using both acupuncture and one of the manipulative therapies in tandem is best of all: acupuncture is used to relax the often crippling muscular spasms and manipulation can address the underlying mechanical or postural problem. The good news for sufferers is that relief is usually swift and 70 to 80 per cent of patients with acute back pain feel better after two or three sessions of either therapy.

MANIPULATIVE THERAPIES

If you are suffering from back pain, and looking to try just one treatment, the evidence indicates that manipulative therapies should be your first choice as they often cure the existing problem.

The evidence for the success of these therapies has been proven in some good clinical trials.

● The most comprehensive study ever attempted was organized at Northwick Hospital in 1990. Chiropractic and conventional hospital methods were compared. A total of 741 patients were randomly allocated treatment from either approach. Chiropractic was significantly more successful in alleviating acute (short-term) back pain than the conventional hospital methods (physiotherapy and painkillers). Two years later a significant number of the chiropractic patients were still pain-free [1].

● At least two studies show patients who receive either osteopathy or chiropractic return to work twice as fast as those being treated by Western methods [2].

If you are suffering from acute back pain, two or three sessions with an osteopath or chiropractor are usually needed. If the complaint is chronic (long-term), then more sessions are usually necessary and 'maintenance' treatment to prevent a further attack is recommended particularly if the back pain is aggravated by work. If there is absolutely no improvement after four to six treatments, then manipulative treatment will probably not be the answer for you.

ACUPUNCTURE

The case for acupuncture in the treatment of back pain is not as clear cut as for the manipulative therapies, some studies found that it did very little, but many people have found it very helpful, particularly for pain relief, and there is ample evidence that you should consider it.

● A 1983 study compared acupuncture with a common Western management procedure – an injection with lignocaine (the most commonly used local anaesthetic). Back pain reduction was reduced by 36 per cent for the acupuncture group and 22 per cent for the lignocaine group. The patients who were managed with lignocaine were also subjected to 'random' needling. This means that needles were inserted in areas which were not recognized acupuncture points, thus eliminating the argument that the acupuncture patients' more positive response was down to the 'placebo effect' (3). Another trial in 1975 showed that acupuncture had a greater analgesic (pain-killing) effect than random needling, producing results in one week (4).

● A 1982 study divided 44 patients with back problems into two treatment groups. One group were given acupuncture, the other had treatment by pinching the skin near to the recognized acupuncture point. There was a clear improvement in the acupuncture group: 16 (72 per cent) of the patients in the treatment group were pain-free one month after the completion of treatment compared with five (22 per cent) of the random group who were also pain-free, presumably due to the placebo effect (5).

If there is no improvement after four or five sessions, acupuncture is unlikely to provide long-term relief. Therapists' experience shows that if the back pain has been a persistent problem, then acupuncture will alleviate the pain for around six to nine months, reduce inflammation and promote healing. For the story of a patient who received acupuncture for back pain see page 92.

BOWEL DISEASES

Conventional medical treatment for bowel problems such as ulcerative colitis, Crohn's disease and irritable bowel syndrome (IBS) suppress the symptoms but cannot offer a cure. Many patients are understandably not keen to continue taking long-term medication with no guarantee that they will eventually be clear of the illness.

Complementary medicine can prove very useful when it is combined with conventional medicine. In some cases a cure is possible and even though symptoms do tend to recur with these conditions, a relapse can hold less fear for patients if they have discovered a method of coping with the attacks.

Inflammatory bowel disease (IBD)

The two inflammatory diseases of the bowel where complementary medicine has most to offer are ulcerative colitis and Crohn's disease. The cause of both is unknown, but both produce similar symptoms.

- Diarrhoea.
- Severe abdominal pain.
- Malnourishment – the patient often goes off food completely, coupled with the fact that the gut doesn't absorb food properly – and this can lead to extreme fatigue.
- Blood is sometimes passed from the rectum, particularly in older people. Occasionally blood transfusions might prove necessary.

Ulcerative colitis, however, is primarily restricted to the large intestine and affects the most superficial layers of the gut wall, whereas Crohn's disease predominantly affects the small intestine and all the layers of the gut wall are involved.

Diagnosis for these diseases is usually by sigmoidoscopy (a tube is passed into the bowel so that doctors can take a look at it). Once diagnosis is made, conventional treatment is usually with steroids or sulphasalazine (a drug related to the aspirin family), but these drugs can cause side effects. Surgery to remove part of the bowel is sometimes carried out, but there can be complications with this and there is no guarantee that even after surgery, the symptoms will disappear forever.

Where to start?

The complementary medicine approach in both ulcerative colitis and Crohn's disease is similar and is aimed at the following.

● Restoring the proper function of the gut by testing for and treating dysbiosis.
● Discovering any existing sensitivities to particular foods which could be leading to the inflammation.

A clinical ecologist should be consulted first to discover any food sensitivities and a nutritional therapist may be able to help with diet advice and nutritional supplementation if needed.

Both of these approaches are not usually considered by most British doctors, although in Germany and other parts of Europe they have been established for some time now.

Acupuncture, homoeopathy and hypnosis have all been known to help with the treatment of bowel diseases, although there is as yet no clear clinical evidence to prove this to be true.

DYSBIOSIS

In all our guts live colonies of the so-called 'friendly' bacteria which help our digestive and immune systems to work properly. To generalize, there are two types of bacteria: coliform organisms and lactic acid fermenters. They exist in a balanced way, but a change in diet can alter this balance as can antibiotics or an attack of diarrhoea Signs that dysbiosis is present is a change in bowel action, flatulence and a swollen abdomen.

It is suspected that dysbiosis can result in a food sensitivity and that this could then cause both irritable and inflammatory bowel diseases.

CLINICAL ECOLOGY

A study carried out with 136 Crohn's patients in East Anglia was reported in the Lancet in 1993. They gave up the main foodstuffs known to cause allergic reactions (cows' milk and wheat were the main ones). Of these, 43 failed to carry on with this diet after 14 days; but the 93 who remained were helped by changing their diet: in fact 78 had a complete remission. These patients then stayed on the diet but were given either steroids or placebo drugs. The patients who weren't receiving steroids showed more improvement. They were free of symptoms for seven and a half months – almost double the time that the steroid patients were free of symptoms. Two years later the steroid-free patients were still doing better (1).

It is too early to draw any definite implications about the relevance of steroid treatment but it does show the prime importance of avoiding certain foods in relieving acute attacks of Crohn's disease and staying symptom free.

Excluding certain foods for two to three months may help considerably and avoid the need for powerful drugs.

DESENSITIZATION

It is possible to desensitize patients to their allergies by giving them small amounts of allergic foods by injection, at monthly, then three and six monthly intervals over a period of one or two years. This has been shown to reduce relapses from ulcerative colitis (2). Again a clinical ecologist can advise if this treatment – known as EPD, (enzyme potentiated desensitization) – is suitable for you.

Because IBD patients cannot absorb nutrients as well as healthy people they may become deficient in certain key minerals and vitamins. They are often deficient in zinc and may need replacement therapy for this and other vitamin or mineral supplements.

Irritable bowel syndrome (IBS)

In the normal digestive process coordinated contractions of the gut wall force food through the digestive tract. If these contractions become uncoordinated due to stress, anxiety or as is suspected food sensitivity, then the subsequent spasms cause bouts of diarrhoea and constipation, pain and abdominal bloating can occur – these are the main symptoms of IBS.

These symptoms can also be due to other conditions, notably irritable bowel disease, but once the diagnosis of IBS is made, the patient faces a challenge. Conventional treatment is aimed solely at alleviating the symptoms and the patient faces a lifetime of coping with a condition, which although not life-threatening, is extremely uncomfortable and is likely to reoccur at any time. There is unlikely to be a 'cure' but the patient can be helped greatly by complementary medicine in that he or she can normally find satisfactory ways of managing the illness.

Where to start?

Dietary changes coupled with relaxation techniques, especially hypnotherapy, are the two approaches which should be considered first of all.

Other relaxation therapies have been reported to help IBS, such as acupuncture. The latter can affect the nerve system which controls the gut's contractions. Four or five treatments may be needed before there is any noticeable improvement.

CLINICAL ECOLOGY

A clinical ecologist can advise on dietary changes. Two approaches can be looked at: excluding any foods to which the patient may be allergic and treating any underlying abnormality in the gut bacteria.

In one reported study over 70 per cent of IBS patients got better after following what is sometimes known as the 'stone-age' diet (3) (see box on page 36 for more information).

When other foods were added to their diet obvious triggers of their irritable bowel were recognized, especially milk and wheat. This last is important when you realize that many IBS patients are told to eat more fibre to help their IBS, when actually this can sometimes make things worse.

On an exclusion diet, you can expect to feel better in two to three months. A clinical ecologist can help reintroduce foods after the initial exclusion.

STONE-AGE DIET

The so-called stone-age diet works on the principle that our digestive system has not evolved much since pre-historic times, and that we would live healthier and longer lives if we ate the sort of foods our bodies evolved to cope with. In practice, this means eating a bland diet of plain fish, uncontaminated meat like lamb and vegetables. Stone-age man didn't process farm produce so foods like wheat and grains aren't included. Fruit would have been a rare treat and only limited kinds would have been available, so you should only eat them in moderate quantities.

HYPNOTHERAPY

This therapy can greatly help to reduce attacks of IBS. The approach to IBS was developed by Dr Peter Whorwell at the Whittington Hospital in Manchester, in fact in one study hypnotherapy achieved an overall 80 per cent improvement in the ailment with patients under 50 achieving a 100 per cent success rate (4). Patients' bowel symptoms, pain and general wellbeing all improved. The results were dramatic and were far superior to the response that was demonstrated from giving the patients a placebo.

Dr Whorwell's approach was to explain the gut's anatomy and functioning to the patients and then under hypnosis to ask them to imagine their bowel acting normally. This 'gut directed hypnosis' got results after four to six sessions. (For the story of one patient who undertook hypnosis for IBS see pages 135–136).

HOMOEOPATHY

Classical homoeopathy has had some success with IBS although there are no clinical trials that report on treatment. Remedies which might be tried to cope with attacks include the following.

Symptom	Remedy
For flatulence, constipation alternating with diarrhoea and pain in the upper left abdomen.	Argent Nit

For burning pains, thirst, frequent
need to urinate, nausea and vomiting and
possibly cystitis.   Cantharis
For gripping stomach pains which double
the patient over.   Colocynth

In a clinical trial a complex homoeopathic treatment using celandine relieved nearly all symptoms in a group of 30 patients over a four-week period. Patients given a placebo did not get any better (5).

CANCER

This is a disease of the cells. New cells are generated daily by the body, some prove to be defective and are normally dealt with by the immune system. However, if they are not detected they can rapidly multiply and develop into a tumour or cancer which attacks healthy tissue. The most common cancer for men is cancer of the lungs and prostate; for women it is breast cancer followed by ovarian, cervical and uterine. There is no known 'cure' for cancer, although many go into remission for years. The outcome of any therapeutic measure, whether conventional or complementary, can never be fully guaranteed. However, some patients find complementary medicine can help them cope with pain and the side effects of conventional treatment, particularly the sickness that follows chemotherapy. In some cases, it has benefited patients who had 'reached the end of the road' with conventional treatment.

This said, there is no clear answer to the question 'how much can complementary medicine help the cancer patient?' What is clear is that many of the brightest and best cancer doctors in the country are increasingly integrating complementary medicine techniques with their own conventional treatment. The impact of this sea-change in opinion should not be underestimated; only 10 to 15 years ago, cancer specialists tended to dismiss complementary medicine as quackery. In the future, it seems increasingly likely that conventional and complementary medicine will work together to help patients tackle and cope with the disease.

Until we find the cure for cancer (if such a thing is ever possible), complementary therapy offers something which conventional medicine does not. When there is no hope left, it can support patients in their efforts to face up to the end of their lives with dignity. If, as has been said, 'the challenge of life is not just to live well, but to die well', complementary medicine is our best tool – it nourishes the spirit, gives a sense of control back to the patient and helps in ways which we may never be able to explain adequately.

This sense of control is an important one. Patients whose conventional treatment was supplemented with complementary medicine have benefited greatly by the feeling that they are doing something to help themselves. The effects this has on the healing process are still being examined but are likely to prove profound.

Where to start?

There is no obvious therapy to help cancer, but these treatments can give relief, depending on the patient and the form the cancer takes.

Good, well-controlled trials have shown that acupuncture has much to offer. There is also evidence that mind–body therapies can have a positive result. Healing is very successful in calming and focusing patients. Nutritional medicine (including dietary changes) and homoeopathy can also prove useful.

ACUPUNCTURE

Cancer patients report that while being treated in hospital, much of their pain is not due to their disease but relates to the radiotherapy, chemotherapy and the operations they receive. In one study acupuncture was found to provide effective pain relief on a long-term basis for around two-thirds of hospital cancer patients. It helped reduce the pain caused by their treatment but it also helped pain that resulted from spread of the cancer (1).

Acupuncture has also been found useful for reducing the nausea produced by chemotherapy (2). There is one problem, however, the nausea tends to last for around four to five days following treatment, and acupuncture works most effectively if given on a daily basis for this period. Obviously this is not so convenient for the patient. Acupressure bands (Sea-Bands) which stimulate the points have also been found to provide some relief (3), but not to the same degree.

NUTRITIONAL MEDICINE

If you want to improve your chances of *not* developing cancer, there are certain dietary measures that you can take which can help you stay disease free. We still don't know the extent to which these changes can help patients who have already developed cancer, but they do give back to patients a sense of control over their illness.

It has been proven that certain types of diet, particularly those rich in anti-oxidants, can help prevent cancers starting. Cancer results because of damage to the cells' DNA by toxic by-products called free radicals. These can be neutralized by the so-called anti-oxidants; vitamins A, C, E and beta carotene (the plant version of vitamin A).

Much interest has been focused on the idea that vitamin and mineral supplementation could prevent cancer. But there is no clear evidence that vitamin supplements can prevent or fight cancers. What is claimed is that vitamin A, C and E and beta carotene are thought to block the formation of cancer-causing agents and prevent the conversion of some cancer-causing agents into their active forms. They may also act to destroy newly formed cancer cells. Although not yet proven to do any good it may help for cancer patients to take dietary supplements in doses two to three times the recommended minimum daily requirements. See the following table for some useful guidelines.

SUGGESTED DAILY SUPPLEMENT LEVELS OF ANTI-OXIDANTS

	Active cancer	**Maintenance level**
Vitamin A	10 000 IU	7500 IU
Beta carotene	25 000 IU	10 000 IU
Vitamin C	6–10 g	1–3 g
Vitamin E	200–400 IU	100 IU
Selenium	200 µg	100 µg

The maintenance level refers to suggested doses to stay healthy, not the Recommended Daily Allowanaces (RDAs).

(Source: Goodman et al, 1994. J.Nutr Med, 4, 199–214.)

Apparently about 35 per cent of cancers are partly due to poor dietary habits and a contributing factor in one per cent of these is because of additives, pesticides and fertilizers. Claims have been made, notably since the '70s, that following strict diets can actually benefit patients where the disease is established. The pioneer of this approach in Great Britain is the Bristol Cancer Care Centre. For the last 20 years it has been promoting the treatment of cancer via dietary changes. In its early days, the Bristol centre advocated a strict vegan diet, totally dependent on organic produce grown free of pesticides and other chemicals. More recently their advice has been less stringent although they still recommend a vegan diet, with the proviso that the diet fits the patient: some people would not benefit from the vegan regime.

The Centre's approach is to focus on a diet which promotes health and wellbeing. Basically, the salient points of the diet are as follows.

To stick to natural, unprocessed foods. Ideally you should eat and drink daily:

- 3–4 servings of wholegrains (wild and brown rice, barley, oats, millet, rye, wheat and corn).
- 3–4 servings of vegetables, raw or lightly steamed.
- 3–4 servings of fruits rich in vitamin C, particularly citrus such as oranges and grapefruit.
- 1–2 servings of pulses, beans, peas or lentils.
- Sesame, sunflower seeds and nuts should be used as snacks.
- Filtered water is recommended as it is relatively free of chemical or mineral contaminants.

The Bristol Centre recommends avoiding the following:
alcohol, tea, coffee and caffeinated drinks (caffeine affects the digestion, blood pressure and cholesterol as well as reducing the normal absorption of iron and zinc), salt, chemical preservatives, therefore processed foods as much as possible, sugar, saturated fat, hydrogenated margarine, processed polyunsaturated fats and deep-fried foods (these all promote inflammatory reactions), smoking.

These foods should be eaten in only moderation:
eggs, dairy products, such as milk and cheese, fish, white meat.

Other strict diets and fasting regimes (especially the Gerson diet) have generated interest, but there is no clinical proof that these diets do any good long term although there are many such anecdotal reports.

MIND–BODY THERAPIES

Psychoneuroimmunology (PNI) – the study of how our emotions and mind affect our response to disease – is one of the fastest growing branches of medicine. PNI is sure to hold important clues for the future treatment of cancer.

It is known that treatment aimed at supporting patients at vulnerable times can affect the function of the body's 'natural killer' cells whose job it is to destroy cancerous cells. Although research is still in its infancy, it looks as if we are increasingly going to find connections between the working of the brain and emotions and how well our bodies can cope with disease.

One study, of 35 women diagnosed with breast cancer who were followed up over a period of 10 years, showed that those women who showed a fighting spirit and refused to accept their diagnosis as a death sentence lived significantly longer than those who felt hopeless or impotent or even accepted their illness stoically. However, the researchers did not measure the extent of the spread of the disease to the underarm lymph nodes (this is the clearest indicator of how long a breast cancer patient can expect to live). Therefore, we don't know if the women who survived simply did not have as severe a form of the disease when they entered into the study as those who didn't.

The danger of quoting this type of research is that the patients might infer from it that they have either brought on their illness or have hindered their chances of getting better by failing to adopt the right attitude. There is as yet also no evidence that specific emotions or stressful events make a person more likely to get, or recover, from cancer. And we have not proven that there is a certain kind of person who is more prone to get cancer as we have for, say, heart disease.

What we do know is that cancer patients can be significantly helped by the application of what is known as 'psychosocial' medicine. In the famous research carried out by David Spiegel in the 1970s, it was discovered that advanced-stage cancer patients who were offered group therapy along with hypnosis and relaxation training for a year along with their conventional medical care lived 18 months longer than those who only received medical care (4). The original point of the research was to explore if this holistic approach helped to improve the quality of life of end-stage cancer patients – which it certainly did. What surprised Spiegel was that it apparently increased the 'quantity' of life too.

NHS hospitals are increasingly offering some form of psychosocial and mind–body medicine to their patients alongside chemotherapy, surgery and radiotherapy. It has been shown that a combination of aromatherapy, massage, counselling and healing has helped patients regain a sense of control. Support groups are a useful alternative to counselling. A study at the University of California showed that patients who attended social support groups that offered counselling, education and training in stress management were less distressed in just six weeks (5).

Other relaxation techniques to consider include meditation, visualization, hypnosis and a form of mind training known as biofeedback, which helps patients gain control over their involuntary body responses. These help patients with nausea and depression. They also help patients to cope with the fact that even if they go into remission, they will still have to live with the understandable fear of the cancer returning. In addition, as shown by the Spiegel research, they are invaluable in helping those who cannot expect to survive very long to focus on what is important in their life and to make the most of the time that is left to them.

The Bristol Cancer Care Centre has been in the forefront of introducing this 'psychosocial' approach to the UK. They will provide information on the use of mind–body techniques in cancer care. They can be contacted by calling 0117 980 9500.

CANDIDIASIS

Hippocrates wrote about candidiasis (also known as thrush) nearly two and a half thousand years ago and one would think that a disease we have known about for so long would be less of a mystery to us by now. But much is still unclear about candidiasis, including its cause, its diagnosis and ultimately the best form of treatment.

Classic symptoms of candidiasis include a disrupted bowel action, bloating, lethargy and cravings for sugar and carbohydrates. It can also appear in the vagina and also in the mouth or on the skin.

Candidiasis is thought to be due to an overgrowth of a tiny yeast organism, *Candida albicans*, a fungus which is naturally present in all of our guts from shortly after birth. It is only when it gets out of control that it becomes a problem. It is obvious that the presence of the fungus in the gut is a major cause of the abdominal discomfort, but it seems that candida also affects other parts of the body resulting in a whole host of symptoms including diarrhoea, constipation, wind, bloating, abdominal pain, heartburn, anal itching, fatigue, impaired concentration, mood swings, anxiety, irritability, depression, recurrent skin fungal infections, recurrent vaginal or oral thrush, severe menstrual and premenstrual disturbance, recurrent cystitis, catarrh, skin disorders, sugar cravings and multiple food sensitivities.

There are several theories as to how this happens. None of these are proven to be the cause of candidiasis, but all of them may be involved to a greater or lesser degree.

● Candida overgrowth results in a malfunctioning gut ('leaky gut'), and this allows toxins to seep out into the blood and circulate to other parts of the body. A further complication is that these set off an allergic-type response to other foods.

● Candida ferments carbohydrates into alcohol, causing alcohol-related products in the gut, as well as the phenomenon of the patient getting drunk from eating carbohydrates.

Diagnosis for candidiasis is difficult. There is no hard and fast method. People suffering from symptoms consistent with candidiasis usually have to be treated for a couple of months, and if they respond, candidiasis is assumed to be the cause.

Antifungal treatment may well be prescribed by your doctor, coupled with a no-sugar, no-yeast diet plus probiotic therapy (supplementing with friendly bacteria such as *Lactobacillus acidophilus*). Coming off as many drugs as possible is a good idea as these can affect the bacteria in the gut. It has also been suggested that the oral contraceptive pill is linked to the development of candidiasis.

Antifungal treatment with the drug, nystatin, has been shown to be very good at relieving candidiasis. Doctors have reported 'dramatic' improvement and results within about two to four weeks although longer treatment is usually recommended.

One study, however, showed that it wasn't much more use than a placebo (1), but the patients had not been asked to observe the no-sugar, no-yeast rule. At best all that can be assumed from this study is that nystatin is not particularly effective if you keep on eating sugar and yeast.

Nystatin treatment is usually recommended for four to six months, and the no-sugar, no-yeast diet should also be followed for this period, and ideally for longer. If you choose to complement conventional treatment with other measures, you will probably have to see a nutritional therapist once a month after the initial consultation until symptoms clear.

Where to start?

A nutritional therapist can help with the diet and probiotics, and detect any food sensitivity which might be related to the symptoms of candidiasis. Acupuncture can help in boosting a sufferer's weak immune system.

Both homoeopathy and herbalism can also prove helpful in the treatment of candidiasis.

NUTRITIONAL MEDICINE

Vitamin supplementation has been promoted by some therapists as a way of dealing with candidiasis, but no hard proof exists. The same is true of certain herbs that can be used for treatment (see below). Again a nutritional therapist can advise if this would help, and it certainly could do no harm.

No-sugar, no-yeast diet

This is almost certainly advisable for anyone trying to rid themselves of candidiasis. Sugar is its main food and cutting out sugar and refined carbohydrates (sugary foods such as biscuits) 'starves' the fungus. Avoiding foods with a high yeast content (alcohol and bread, for instance) will help sometimes, although this might not be necessary in all patients. Some sufferers, but by no means all, develop a sensitivity whereby the yeast in the food reacts with their candida.

Probiotics
These are concentrated supplements of 'gut friendly' bacteria, for instance *Lactobacillus acidophilus*. Studies have shown that lactobacilli inhibit the growth of candida. Skill is needed to identify the best probiotic for each patient and in determining the level at which the patient should be dosed.

ACUPUNCTURE
This therapy has been reported to be useful, and certainly it makes sense that it should, because acupuncture stimulates a weakened immune system. Therapists' experience is that acupuncture helps, but no trials of acupuncture for treating candidiasis have been reported.

HOMOEOPATHY
Homoeopathy treatment focuses on giving the patient constitutional treatment to help the candida. Specific remedies can also be taken to relieve vaginal and other types of thrush.

HERBALISM
Some herbal treatments have been reported to have good results against candida. The treatment is tailored to the patient.

CHRONIC FATIGUE SYNDROME
How Chronic Fatigue Syndrome (or myalgic encephalomyelitis – ME) develops isn't known, and a 'cure' has still not been found. Some comfort for sufferers of this debilitating condition (and there are estimated to be as many as 200,000 in Britain) is that 80 to 90 per cent of cases do recover in time. But how long it takes to recover can't be predicted, and this coupled with the many symptoms causes sufferers to become anxious and depressed.

CFS or ME – the terms have become synonymous in the last few years – is a controversial disease. Does it really exist or is it a figment of the imagination? That has been asked by almost every newspaper and magazine. The answer is no, it is not a neurotic condition.

Although much is still unknown, CFS sufferers often demonstrate a definite pattern of deficiencies and disorders which point towards it being a definite disease, albeit one that is difficult to diagnose. These include evidence of viral infiltration of the muscles (which would explain the muscular weakness), low magnesium in the red cells and abnormal nutritional and hormonal function.

CFS can be traced back to a viral infection from which the patient never properly recovered. Flu could be to blame, but other viruses, such as herpes and enteroviruses have also been known to cause it; sometimes the sufferer cannot exactly pinpoint the infection. In order to help with diagnosis, Australian researchers developed a table of 'major and supporting signs'.

If two major symptoms together with five of the supporting symptoms are present, this is a sound basis for suspecting CFS.

Major signs of CFS

● Persistent or intermittent periods of fatigue for more than six months, which are made worse by exercise.
● Poor concentration and short-term memory problems or other similar mental impairment.
● Decreased immune response and a reduction in white blood cells (which fight infection) although this may not be the case by the time the patient first consults their doctor and has tests.

Supporting signs

● Muscle pain and tenderness, joint pain, headaches, depression, tinnitus, insomnia, swollen glands, recurrent sore throats and irritable bowel syndrome.

Where to start?

Visiting a nutritional therapist for supplements should be considered by all CFS patients. Acupuncture can improve the patient's immune system and classical and complex homoeopathy can often significantly ease the sufferer's symptoms.

Other therapies that are worth trying include healing, which has been known to help symptoms that are hindering the body's ability to heal, and consulting a clinical ecologist to identify any underlying food intolerances. A large majority of patients find that avoiding specific foods helps, and a general improvement in diet (including avoiding processed and junk foods) works too, presumably by boosting the immune system.

Expect at least seven or eight treatments to be needed before there is significant improvement.

NUTRITIONAL MEDICINE
Seventy-five per cent of all CFS patients have derived benefit from taking nutritional supplements and this is the only therapy that has been proven to work.

Evening primrose oil, if it is taken at the dose of 2 to 3g for two to three months, has helped 70 per cent of patients (1).

CFS patients have been shown to have low magnesium in the red cells and magnesium injections (directly into the muscles) have shown to benefit 70 per cent of such patients (2). Usually between four and eight injections are needed.

Generally the complementary medical approach to CFS is to support the immune system and sometimes to combat the virus directly. There are no clinical trials to back up the following therapies but they have been reported to be useful by therapists and patients.

ACUPUNCTURE
An experienced acupuncturist who follows the traditional Chinese approach should be consulted. The approach is to boost the body's immunity and to strengthen weakened organs. Treatment will have to take place over a prolonged period as the effects will wear off, but the patient should see some improvement after six to 10 sessions.

HOMOEOPATHY
Excellent results using classical homoeopathy have been reported for the treatment of CFS if the right remedy can be matched to the patient profile. One recent controlled trial has shown that clear benefit was felt by patients receiving classical homoeopathy over a period of one year: 60 per cent of the patients improved in the homoeopathy group as opposed to 20 per cent of patients in the placebo group (3).

Complex homoeopathy depends on using small doses of the virus thought to have initiated the illness along with herbal and homoeopathic remedies, targeted to support specific organs which seem to be working least well, frequently the liver and colon in CFS. The liver may also be weakened. This approach is very popular in France and Germany and is gaining popularity here. For the story of a patient treated for CFS with clinical ecology, turn to pages 129–130.

PSYCHOLOGICAL APPROACHES IN CFS

Chronic Fatigue Syndrome is a very complex disease, and as has been pointed out, one we don't fully understand. In recent years, there has been more emphasis on the physical symptoms of the disease. Experts have shied away to some extent from dealing with the psychological symptoms in case this was seen as an implication that CFS was 'all in the mind'. But now the psychological symptoms of the patients are again coming to the fore.

A joint report by the Royal Colleges of Physicians, Psychiatrists and General Practitioners states: 'CFS cannot be considered either physical or psychological – both need to be considered simultaneously to understand the syndrome.'

Some 50 to 70 per cent of sufferers experience depression, anxiety or another psychological disorder. The jury is still out on whether depression arises because of the limitations placed on the patient by CFS or whether it is an intrinsic part of the disease. It could be a combination of both. Either way, it's essential that the patient is supported through this in any way that seems appropriate. Healing and counselling can help. A form of therapy known as cognitive behavioural therapy may be useful (although some experts disagree). Unlike many forms of therapy, with cognitive behavioural therapy, the therapist is 'interactive' as opposed to 'passive': he or she helps the patient look for positive ways of behaving and thinking that alter the way that the patient views the disease and his or her limitations.

Cognitive behavioural therapy can help patients turn around their attitude towards the disease which can give them a great deal of relief. One good example of how this works is in relation to exercise. The exhaustion arising from CFS is a major problem. Patients don't feel able to undertake even the simplest of tasks. Some experts have recommended that patients follow a graded exercise programme as a means of combating this exhaustion whether they feel like it or not. But that approach has now fallen out of favour. The best advice for patients who have the classic symptoms of CFS is to take a period of proper rest, followed by convalescence. They should not rush back into normal activities too soon or they risk a relapse. However, it has been shown to be helpful for patients to start exercising a little each day should they feel up to it. This should be gentle and never forced. They have to learn how to pace their activity and conserve their limited energy supplies and be prepared for some days being worse than others.

Cognitive behavioural therapy, by helping patients to accept their limitations when it comes to exercise, but at the same time still keep trying to expand these limits, may prevent them sinking into an understandable state of hopelessness. This is a natural reaction with a long-term, unpredictable disease like CFS.

DEPRESSION

Depression is a common response to illness, bereavement or general dissatisfaction with life. This sort of depression can be helped by complementary medicine. But severe depression is an illness (so-called 'endogenous' depression) and although this type, too, can be helped by complementary medicine, a doctor should always be consulted first. Symptoms include low self esteem, a severe feeling of emptiness, mood swings, despair and irritability. Antidepressant drugs are usually prescribed; some of the latest such as Prozac have much fewer side effects than older style antidepressants. When depression is severe, it is best to get orthodox treatment as fast as possible while working out a complementary medicine strategy which can work alongside orthodox medicine.

Where to start?

Treatment for depression can often take a long time although sometimes, the patient can respond very quickly. Herbalism has been shown to be just as effective as treatment with the most commonly prescribed antidepressants. Nutritional medicine has also proved to be a useful treatment.

Since sensitivity to foods and chemicals is implicated in depression, ruling out any such allergy by consulting a clinical ecologist may also help enormously. There is some evidence that electroacupuncture works well with depressives. Homoeopathy has also proven successful although there are no clinical studies to back this up. There is no research into healing aiding depression, but it is known to help alleviate feelings of despair brought on by long-term, chronic ill-health and so should be considered.

HERBALISM

St John's Wort (*Hypericum perforatum*) has been found to be extremely useful in treating depression, and is as good as antidepressant drugs at doing so, which has lead to the nickname 'the natural Prozac'. Indeed some studies show that it is more useful than the drugs most often prescribed and doesn't have the side effects (1). Results are usually quick: improvement can be seen in as little as two weeks, with far fewer side effects than conventional antidepressants.

Another herb *Ginkgo biloba* has been found to lift depression when used in conjunction with antidepressants in patients who had not before responded well to antidepressant drugs (2).

NUTRITIONAL MEDICINE

Deficiencies of many of the B vitamins have been implicated in patients suffering from depression. Improvement has been seen in the patients that are given folic acid, riboflavin and pyridoxine (3). The latter is crucial for depressed women who are taking the contraceptive pill (4). Out of 39 depressed women on the Pill, 19 were deficient in pyridoxine. When given supplements of it, 16 got better.

Vitamin C therapy at a dose of 1g daily improved the depression of some patients in three weeks (5). (It has been suggested that some depression is linked to vitamin C deficiency as patients respond well to eating far more fruit and vegetables than they would normally.) Other possible supplements are magnesium and evening primrose oil.

CLINICAL ECOLOGY

Food and chemical sensitivity can be important causes of depression. It has been shown that patients with severe psychiatric illness responded well when they avoided certain foods to which they proved sensitive (6). Depressed people have a higher than average likelihood of being allergic to various triggers. In one study of 109 depressed children, 85 per cent of them were 'allergic types'. It has even been suggested that the reason some antidepressant drugs work so well is that they are potent antihistamines (7).

ACUPUNCTURE

Electroacupuncture has proved to be as effective as some anti-depressants and is thought to work by acting on nervous system chemical transmitters (8). In another study, when 30 patients were treated in some cases for as long as four months, and sometimes daily, 25 of them showed improvement and 13 were cured completely (9).

HOMOEOPATHY

There are no clinical studies to back it up, but homoeopaths report good results for depression if the patient profile can be matched successfully with the remedy. Here are some of the most commonly prescribed treatments.

Symptom	Remedy
For when the patient feels under a black cloud and is potentially suicidal.	Aurum metallicum
For when patients cry but not in public.	Natrum muriaticum
For when there is depression along with anger.	Nux vomica
For when patient is upset easily and resentful.	Staphisagria
For when there is a feeling of 'I just don't care'.	Sulphur

HAY FEVER

Hay fever is the allergic reaction to airborne allergens (usually pollen during spring and summer) but it is rarely caused by just one trigger. Symptoms include a runny nose, sneezing, red, itchy eyes and a sore throat. Conventional medicine blocks the action of histamine (see diagram on page 52) with antihistamine drugs and with inhalers which widen the air passages allowing the sufferer to breathe more easily. Complementary medicine is aimed at identifying, avoiding and desensitizing the body to the allergens as well as strengthening any underlying weaknesses which may be contributing to the allergy.

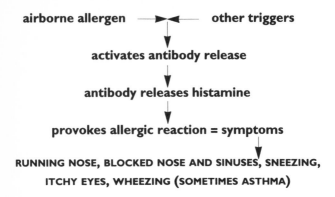

Where to start?

As has been said above, pollen is the main allergic cause of hay fever-like symptoms, but hay fever is rarely triggered by just one allergen. It makes sense to consult a clinical ecologist to determine if anything else is contributing to the discomfort, and for possible desensitization treatment. Homoeopathy has also had very good results in improving hay fever symptoms. Treatment should always be started at least two months before the main hay fever season begins.

Nutritional medicine strengthens the cell walls of histamine-releasing cells so they don't 'explode' so easily. Acupuncture and herbal medicine can also strengthen the immune system.

WHAT CAN CAUSE YOUR HAY FEVER?	
Months when symptoms are worse	**Likely allergen**
February – May	trees
June – July	grass
July – August	nettles, mugwort, golden rod
late July – autumn	mould, fungus

CLINICAL ECOLOGY

There is a commonly held, but as yet unproven, view among complementary therapists that food allergies make the symptoms of hay fever worse. Identifying and cutting out these foods means there is a reduction in the hay fever symptoms. If you're careful to avoid these foods, the hay fever symptoms can clear completely. If this is so, it means that the allergic symptoms weren't caused by pollen in the first place but to foods eaten only in summer, or in larger quantities in summer.

When the symptoms are due to food you will find they get worse immediately on chewing the food, or around six to 10 hours after eating it, and sometimes as much as 24 hours after eating.

However, it has to be said that the vast majority of hay fever sufferers are allergic to airborne allergens. But again, more than just pollen can be the trigger. Other 'culprits' can also identified and these include cigarette smoke, perfume, industrial pollutants and air pollution from car fumes. Sulphur dioxide may cause problems – in very rare cases wine, beer, cider and dried fruits may act as triggers as these are preserved in sulphur compounds. Take-away fast food can also set off symptoms as the chips used in the fast food industry are often dipped in a sulphur compound.

All the well-known allergens (such as house dust mites, damp places and pets) can work in conjunction with pollen to encourage hay fever symptoms and measures can be taken to minimize their effect.

Once the true allergen picture has been worked out, the clinical ecologist can desensitize the patient (see pages 124–130).

HOMOEOPATHY

The treatments given in homoeopathy have been found to be very helpful in reducing discomfort in hay fever sufferers.

In fact, in one study, 144 patients given remedies of mixed grass pollens had far fewer symptoms, which was proven by the fact that they needed 50 per cent less antihistamine medication (1).

The more 'classical' approach to homoeopathy – where the patient profile is matched to the remedy – is also successful. Some of the remedies known to help include the following.

Symptom	Remedy
For sneezing and when the nose is running.	Natrum mur
For when there are also headaches.	Agaricus
For when there is nasal obstruction and pain above the eyes.	Pulsatilla
For when catarrh is yellow or white and stringy.	Kali bich
For sore nasal bones and depression.	Aurum metallicum

NUTRITIONAL MEDICINE

For certain individuals, nutritional medicine can be very useful to relieve their hay fever symptoms.

In one study, it was discovered that when vitamin C levels dropped to below 1 mg per 100ml of blood, histamine levels rose steeply (2) and when 11 patients with low vitamin C levels were given 1mg of vitamin C for three days, their histamine levels dropped down. In another study, 60 patients were either given vitamin C in a low dose or a high dose (along with thiamine, another vitamin). Fifty per cent of the patients on the lower dose and 75 per cent on the higher dose reported that their symptoms had improved (3).

Supplements of vitamin E were given to patients for five to seven days and proved successful in reducing the actions of histamine (4). Bioflavonoids, nutrients that are found naturally in orange pith, lemons and green peppers, also help to inhibit histamine release (5).

A nutritional therapist can advise on diagnosing any deficiencies the patient is suffering and treating them appropriately.

ACUPUNCTURE

There are no clinical studies to back up acupuncture for treating hay fever but acupuncturists report good results. At least six treatments will be needed each summer to show any improvement in treating patients afflicted by hay fever.

HERBAL MEDICINE

Herbal treatments have been found to be extremely succesful in reducing the symptoms of hay fever sufferers. In one study of 69 patients who stuck with the treatment programme, a remedy of stinging nettles was found to be more successful than a placebo in treating all their hay fever symptoms (6).

HORMONAL AND FERTILITY PROBLEMS
Premenstrual syndrome (PMS)

PMS is a general term for many different symptoms that women may experience together or singly every month between the time of ovulation and the start of their period. Some symptoms are physical in nature, others are more emotional or behavioural. The main symptoms of PMS include irritability, anxiety, depression, fatigue, food cravings, fluid retention and breast enlargement and tenderness, abdominal bloating, clumsiness and poor concentration. Some women suffer badly with many symptoms of PMS, while others experience only a few and even report additional energy and sexual enjoyment during this phase.

The root cause of PMS symptoms is thought to be an irregularity in the finely tuned balance between the hormones oestrogen and progesterone throughout the menstrual cycle. Orthodox medicine treats it by regulating hormones via the contraceptive pill. The other approach is to treat individual symptoms by prescribing, for example, diuretics for water retention and mild tranquillizers for anxiety.

Where to start?

The most widely researched complementary medicine for PMS is nutritional medicine and it has proven positive effects. Acupuncture is a good second choice to nutritional medicine and in some cases, herbal medicine and clinical ecology can help.

NUTRITIONAL MEDICINE
Most people suffering from PMS will benefit significantly from nutritional medicine treatment.

Vitamin B6: several studies have shown that supplementation with this vitamin is significantly better than a placebo at reducing the symptoms of PMS. Water retention is one symptom of PMS that doesn't respond particularly well to such treatment, but vitamin B6 has been shown to help reduce the amount of weight that water-retaining women put on by about an average of 1.4 kg (3 lb). Doses prescribed ranged between 100 to 500 mg daily and the women took the supplement for a period of approximately 3 months (1, 2). In another study vitamin B6 was given to women who were also on the oral contraceptive pill. They took 50mg daily at the first sign of PMS symptoms. Most women reported some improvement. Too much vitamin B6 can also cause PMS but taking 50 to 100mg daily is a safe but effective dose (3).

Vitamin E: two months treatment with natural vitamin E has been shown to help relieve anxiety, food cravings and depression symptoms of PMS. Water retention, however, did not respond as well to this particular supplement (4).

Magnesium: low magnesium in red blood cells is thought to be associated with the anxiety symptoms of PMS and it may also cause the food cravings. In one study of 192 patients, magnesium was given for one week premenstrually and two days during menstruation. Tension was relieved in 89 per cent of patients, breast tenderness in 96 per cent, weight gain was less in 95 per cent, and headaches were reduced in 43 per cent (5).

Evening primrose oil: this has proven to be very useful if taken at a dose of 1,000mg three times a day for a period of two to three months. All of the symptoms responded well but reduction in water retention was treated the least successfully of them. However, irritability, depression and breast tenderness did respond particularly well to this treatment (6, 7).

ACUPUNCTURE

There are no clinical trials to prove how well acupuncture can treat the symptoms of PMS, but it is often used very successfully to treat the condition. It works by regulating the hormonal balance.

HERBAL MEDICINE

Herbal treatments can often help to reduce PMS symptoms. One particular remedy is a herb called Vitex which affects the balance of oestrogen and progesterone leading to a reduction in PMS symptoms. In a survey of 1,542 women, over 90 per cent of cases were helped by this treatment (8).

CLINICAL ECOLOGY

This therapy has been found to be very helpful in treating PMS. In fact, studies have shown that some women may be 'allergic' to their own hormones with the reproductive organs being the 'target' (9). Patients can be treated with dilutions of specific hormones to desensitize them – the so-called 'provocative neutralization' technique – with great success (10). The experience of the team at the University of Southampton is that desensitizing not with oestrogen and progesterone but with the hormones which cause their release, namely prolactin, FSH and LH, works much better in relieving the symptoms of PMS.

Certain foods are known to aggravate PMS symptoms and should be avoided or reduced to gain relief.

Caffeine drinks make a huge difference to PMS: in one study 61 per cent of patients drinking between 4 and 15 caffeine drinks a day suffered moderate to severe symptoms while only 16 per cent of those not drinking caffeinated drinks suffered from PMS (11).

Sugar intake is significantly greater in women who suffer from PMS and cutting down on sugary products three days prior to menstruation can significantly improve the symptoms experienced (12). Salt intake, if it is reduced at least three days prior to menstruation, can also reduce water retention and food cravings (13). If PMS sufferers cut down the amount of milk and dairy products consumed it can help reduce symptoms associated with anxiety (14). (Patients with anxiety have also been shown to eat more dairy products than normal.)

HOMOEOPATHY

There are no clinical trials to prove the benefits of homoeopathy with PMS, but the following have been used successfully in its treatment.

Symptom	Remedy
For breast tenderness.	Calcaria
For irritability.	Causticum
For weight increase.	Graphites
For fluid retention and breast heaviness.	Lachesis
For irritability and anger.	Nux vomica
For weepiness.	Pulsatilla
For depression, irritability and reduced sex drive.	Sepia

Menopause

The menopause is defined in medical terms as the end of menstruation. The average age women reach the menopause is 51, but the time leading up to the menopause (the climacteric) lasts for about 10 to 15 years during which a woman's ovaries slowly stop producing oestrogen. The symptoms of the menopause, which include 'hot flushes', night sweats, depression and lack of sex drive can be very distressing. The accompanying decrease in circulation of the hormone oestrogen in the blood also puts post-menopausal women at higher risk of osteoporosis (bone thinning). In recent years, hormone replacement therapy (HRT) has had a huge amount of media coverage and achieved a certain popularity for treating the menopause, but many women are wary of taking artificial hormones on a long-term basis, and would probably be more interested in taking a natural substitute for HRT.

Where to start?

Nutritional medicine is the best researched and the surest method for treating menopausal symptoms for most women.

Acupuncture treatment can reduce menopausal symptoms, and herbal medicine and clinical ecology may provide some benefit. Homoeopathic remedies may also give some relief to the symptoms.

NUTRITIONAL MEDICINE

This therapy is the most successful in helping menopausal women. When a nutritional therapist is consulted, supplementation will be geared to the individual patient, but treatment will probably be combined with various combinations of those supplements already recommended for PMS (see pages 55– 56).

ACUPUNCTURE
Acupuncture can help with the balance of hormones in the same way it helps with PMS.

HERBAL MEDICINE
Herbal treatments are generally very safe to use and can be a good choice to alleviate menopausal symptoms which can continue for several years. Herbs containing phyto-oestrogens are a good option and they include: dong quai, liquorice root, panax ginseng and black cohosh. The latter has been shown in numerous studies to combat oestrogen deficiency and is a good natural substitute for HRT (1). Natural progesterones, found for instance in wild yams, can also help relieve menopausal symptoms.

CLINICAL ECOLOGY
Women who are suffering from menopausal symptoms may be sensitive to their own hormones as outlined for PMS.

HOMOEOPATHY
Homeopathic remedies can help to adjust the imbalance in a woman's body during the menopause. There have been no clinical trials to prove how successful homoeopathy is, but the following are among the treatments which have been used successfully.

Symptom	Remedy
For hot flushes and depression.	Aurum met
For hot sweats, back ache and dragging sensations.	Sepia
For flushes which are worse at night, and weariness.	Sulphuric acid
For when there is a tendency to gain weight.	Graphites

INFERTILITY PROBLEMS

For couples who are trying to conceive, the news that they are unlikely ever to do so can be devastating. As everyone knows in recent years orthodox medicine has made great leaps in helping these couples, but complementary medicine can act as good support to orthodox fertility treatment, maximizing its chances of working, and even proving successful in some cases where orthodox medicine has failed. Both partners should consider nutritional medicine. Deficiencies in nutrients key to fertility, especially selenium and zinc, when given in supplements can have dramatically good results. An organization called Foresight has been quietly treating fertility problems nutritionally for years, often very successfully.

Foresight doctors sometimes call on Traditional Chinese Medical (TCM) practitioners to work alongside them. Chinese tradition treats infertility in a number of ways. Herbs are usually the main treatment as they generally work faster than acupuncture at treating 'phlegm' conditions. Phlegm conditions include disorders like ovarian cysts and other causes of pelvic inflammatory disease (PID) which affect a woman's fertility.

Acupuncture is also used to help restore hormonal balance and shift Chi (the body's energy) in a more positive way. The treatment is geared to the individual patient and it can work for endometriosis and other forms of PID.

TCM is also useful for patients who are waiting for the start of a fertility programme at a hospital unit. It can strengthen the system and prepare the body for orthodox treatment.There have been cases of women having TCM six months prior to starting fertility treatment who have been able to withdraw from the programme because they have become pregnant without any artificial aid.

While a patient is undergoing IVF (in vitro fertilization) or other hormonal treatments, TCM can help regulate hormones and generally strengthen the woman's system.

It would be wrong to raise false hopes but certainly doctors who work with Foresight, and patients who have used TCM successfully in conjunction with IVF, are very enthusiastic about the potential of complementary medicine to help. The story of one Foresight patient can be found on page 119.

(You can contact Foresight (Pre-conceptual Care) by writing to 28 The Paddock, Godalming, Surrey, GU7 1XB. Enclose a SAE.)

DYSMENORRHOEA (PAINFUL PERIODS)

Painful periods are a source of dread each month. They can be caused by the woman producing too high a level of prostaglandins (hormone-like substances that stimulate womb contractions) but a doctor should always be consulted to check there is no other serious underlying problem, such as a blood or thyroid deficiency, endometriosis, fibroids or a pelvic inflammatory disease. Symptoms of painful periods include cramping, headaches and nausea. Painful periods are mainly treated with painkillers or the contraceptive pill.

The two complementary therapies that should be considered by anyone with painful periods are nutritional therapy and acupuncture. Deficiencies of magnesium, essential fatty acids, calcium and vitamin B6 have all been implicated in dysmenorrhoea. A nutritional therapist can check for individual deficiencies in the patient. Long-term treatment with acupuncture will strengthen the system sufficiently so that the symptoms are lessened or completely cured. Top-ups may be necessary from time to time. If you feel strong enough to undergo acupuncture treatment while suffering a painful period, it may very well take away the pain given its excellent painkilling potential.

Homoeopathy and herbalism can also prove helpful, but treatment is likely to be longer term.

HYPERACTIVITY

Hyperactive children can demonstrate a whole range of abnormal behavioural symptoms: disobedience, poor attention, irritability, aggressiveness, continuous talking, permanent fidgeting, difficulty in making friends, disturbed sleep, poor appetite, attention seeking. Boys suffer from it far more than girls. In babies symptoms of hyperactivity include: colic, lengthy screaming and head-banging.

The mother of a six-year-old hyperactive child has described it as hell: 'There is no relief except when Max is asleep. Even when he's at school, I am always waiting for that dreaded call from the headmistress to say that he is disrupting the class and that I have to come and pick him up'.

Explanations for the condition include reactions to additives in food, and food intolerance. This research is borne out by a study carried out by the Hyperactive Children's Support Group in 1987 which found that there was a high degree of migraine, eczema and asthma in the children's families, suggesting that they are prone to allergy and sensitivity of various sorts. The implication is that hyperactivity is also a sensitivity-disease.

There is a lot of good research that shows there is a definite link between what a child eats and hyperactivity. Studies point to sugar and sugary foods as a major cause of hyperactivity and the experience of doctors working at The Centre for the Study of Complementary Medicine at Southampton in Great Britain confirms this. The worst behaved hyperactive children benefit the most from cutting out sugar. Caffeine, in cola drinks, should also be avoided.

Obviously, life would be easier for both hyperactive children and their parents if they did not have to maintain a strict diet all of the time. It is possible to desensitize children so that they can eat moderate amounts of the foods to which they are allergic. A paper in the Lancet (1) showed that giving children small amounts of the food by injection at two monthly intervals means that they can tolerate foods to which they were previously sensitive.

The Miller technique is another method of desensitizing children (2). A clinical ecologist can advise you on the best way forward (see pages 124–130).

Where to start?

A clinical ecologist or nutritional therapist should be consulted to identify any foods to which your child is sensitive. The therapist will need to carry out the food testing and then recommend a suitable elimination diet where the offending foods are avoided. The testing is accurate in 70 per cent of cases and food elimination is successful in about 70 per cent of these children.

Homoeopathy is also a useful therapy which can help in the treatment of hyperactivity.

CLINICAL ECOLOGY

There are several factors implicated in causing hyperactivity, including learned behaviour patterns and poisoning from lead pipes. However, many hyperactive children are often found to react badly to certain foods, commonly dairy products and food additives. Pinpointing and then avoiding these foods can help greatly, and a clinical ecologist can assist in this.

Avoiding the foods will cut down on the hyperactivity but this is obviously difficult for children and parents. It is possible to desensitize children to the foods to which they are sensitive. This is done by injecting them with small quantities of the food every couple of months. A recent paper in the Lancet showed this to be a highly effective treatment (see page 62).

NUTRITIONAL MEDICINE

This is one of the best therapies to treat hyperactivity as vitamin or mineral deficiencies and food sensitivities can be identified. Hyperactive children have been shown to be deficient in a number of key nutrients and can benefit from being given supplements.

● **Zinc:** hyperactive children excrete large amounts of zinc after eating a food to which they are intolerant, particularly sugar, cola drinks and chocolate. The food colorant tartrazine reduces zinc in the body. Supplementing zinc at bedtime in the form of zinc citrate (the best absorbed zinc salt) is recommended (15mg for young children, and 50mg for children who are six or older) along with a multi B group vitamin which helps zinc absorption.

● **Evening primrose oil**: prostaglandin E1 is one link on a chemical chain which is essential for proper working of the immune system. In hyperactive children it is suspected that PGE1's production is low. Hyperactive children respond very successfully to supplementation with evening primrose oil, which 'steps in' to replace the missing PGE1 on the chemical chain. The children who benefit most are those who have a family history of allergy problems related to the immune system, such as asthma.

HOMOEOPATHY

Mixed medications of herbs and homoeopathic remedies (complex homoeopathy approach) are used to treat hyperactivity and this is often very successful. The Centre for Complementary Medicine at Southampton use traditional Chinese methods to strengthen key organs, especially the pancreas.

Classical homoeopathy (using single remedies) is useful in about 50 per cent of hyperactive cases.

MIGRAINE

When a headache is very severe and may be accompanied by nausea, vomiting and sensory or visual disturbances this is known as a migraine. There are some very good conventional drugs available to help migraine sufferers but even the best ones tend to act by suppressing the symptoms, not curing the cause. For those for whom the drugs do not work, or who suffer frequent attacks, or who do not want to be on drugs long-term, a form of complementary medicine is the natural choice.

The aim is, not just to treat the symptoms, but to get to the root cause of the migraine. There is no ideal therapy, as such, because there are various different underlying reasons for migraine and that determines the best treatment choice. But the following are some of the options worth exploring. To a certain extent you will have to play detective to find out what suits you best.

Do you think your migraine
is linked to food allergy?

Migraine is triggered by certain foods. Approximately 85 per cent of the migraine sufferers who find their trigger foods and exclude them from their diet can keep migraine at bay for long periods (1, 2).

Most people know that migraine can be triggered by chocolate, cheese and coffee, but a great many other foods can set off an attack. Other foods linked to migraine are those containing tyramine (a naturally occurring chemical which acts on nervous system); see page 66 for a list of the common foods containing tyramine.

The list is long, and it can be somewhat daunting to think that all of these foods have to be avoided completely. In reality, the situation isn't quite so dire. Each migraine sufferer has their own individual tolerance to tyramine. A certain amount can be tolerated in a day, but when their own individual 'cut off' point is reached, a migraine develops. Foods contain different concentrations of tyramine and the migraine sufferer can eat tyramine foods to a moderate degree without necessarily having an attack. The tyramine builds up slowly in the body until the 'trigger point' is reached. However, an attack can also be precipitated at levels below the trigger point by other known migraine factors such as too much alcohol or stress.

Most of the studies that have shown food exclusion to be successful, started with the patients following very restrictive diets – primarily eating lamb, pears, fish and vegetables, foods which don't precipitate allergic reactions – and then gradually introducing other foods. Trigger foods are identified when they cause migraine.

This is the 'classical' method of food exclusion. An easier method is to follow an exclusion diet for eight weeks. The key foods known to be the most common 'triggers': milk, cheese, coffee, tea, orange juice, tomatoes, potatoes, chocolate and red wine are all excluded.

After two weeks, and over the following six weeks, reintroducing these foods one at a time will isolate the patient's trigger foods. Eating a trigger food will result in a migraine, usually within 24 hours and it usually proves easy to pinpoint the problem foods.

When trigger foods are isolated and excluded for a long period of time, the patient becomes more tolerant to them and can sometimes eat a small amount without having a migraine.

TYRAMINE-RICH FOODS
(in decreasing order of tyramine concentration starting with cheese
and ending with avocado)

cheese, marmite and other yeast extracts, hard sausage and salami, broad beans, beer, wine (especially red wine), pickled herrings, chocolate, beef, liver, spinach, oranges, prunes, canned meats, figs, hung game, soy sauce, eggs, plums, bananas, tomatoes, pepperoni, aubergines, avocados.

Is your migraine linked to stress, or do you have high blood pressure or insomnia?

Stress is a well-known trigger of migraine. Most of us these days lead stressful lives but it is how we cope with our stress levels that is important, and therapists, from their experience of treating patients, report that often migraine sufferers are the sort of personalities (perfectionists or driven people) who find it hard to relax.

All of the techniques covered in the chapter on mind–body therapies (see pages 130–140) may have something to offer the migraine sufferers. In one study migraine sufferers were given fairly basic relaxation advice on coping with stress and followed up over three years. All of them reported a clear improvement in migraine attacks (3).

Hypnosis has been shown to be more useful than drugs and placebo in one study (4). Meditation and visualization techniques on a daily basis or when an attack is likely because of a particularly stressful period, can also help.

Does your job strain your neck or back? Is your neck stiff and/or is neck and back pain linked with migraine?

Osteopaths and chiropractors both report that manipulative techniques can help reduce migraine although more research is needed. It makes sense that if the neck is stiff and not very mobile, then reducing the tension will cut down on the headaches.

A study of 85 migraine patients given chiropractic or osteopathy showed that they benefited from it (5). There is no evidence that either has the edge over the other (see box on page 100 for help).

ACUPUNCTURE

This is also good for treating migraine, although the evidence is somewhat ambiguous. However, 60 per cent of patients who go for acupuncture experience short-term benefits and some long-term relief. At least six sessions are needed to make a difference and the sustained benefit usually lasts for about a year to a year and a half before more treatment is needed (6).

HOMOEOPATHY

There has been one excellent study which showed that homoeopathy can be dramatically successful in decreasing the frequency, intensity and length of migraine attacks (7). Sixty patients with migraine had their case history taken and were given medication four times over a two-week period. Half the patients' medication was placebo, the other half were given one of eight commonly prescribed homoeopathic treatments for migraine (depending on their profile). Those given the real treatment showed more improvement and needed less medication to control attacks over the four-month follow-up period.

Some of the homoeopathic remedies known to help in migraine, if the patient profile matches, include the following.

Symptom	Remedy
For a 'bursting headache'.	Belladonna
If the migraine is better for staying still.	Bryonia
For a throbbing headache, sometimes brought on by being in the sun.	Glonoine
If you are better being in the open air.	Pulsatilla
For a 'shooting, electric' type of pain.	Magnesium phos.

HERBAL MEDICINE

These remedies can help to relieve migraine, particularly prescription of the herb feverfew. Several studies show that taking this herb regularly decreases the number of attacks and also their ferocity compared with a placebo. Feverfew isn't just taken to combat an attack, it has to be taken daily to have significant effects. However, feverfew appears to have no known side effects.

(See pages 110–111 for details of how one patient was treated for migraine with herbal medicine).

SKIN DISORDERS
Acne

Acne is the most common of all skin problems and affects mainly adolescents and young adults. Generally red, angry spots appear on the skin but acne can also appear as blackheads, whiteheads, pustules and pus-filled cysts. It is a condition linked to the overproduction of sebum (a mixture of oils and waxes) produced by the sebaceous glands in the skin, which lubricates and prevents loss of water from the skin's surface. Sebaceous glands are concentrated on the face and to a lesser extent on the back, shoulders and chest, and these are the areas that are most afflicted. Acne is most common in males. This is because male hormones such as testosterone stimulate the sebaceous glands. There is an increase of male hormones in puberty, in both sexes, which is why the onset of acne afflicts both girls and boys particularly in their teens.

Acne occurs because of a complex interaction between the sebaceous glands, hormones and bacteria, and this interaction can be affected by other factors. For instance, investigations show that 50 per cent of patients with severe acne had increased blood levels of toxins absorbed from the intestines (1). Toxins have been shown to disrupt the copper-zinc ratio and this causes skin inflammation. The toxins may be there in the first place because of a condition called dysbiosis (abnormal gut fermentation) coupled possibly with candidiasis ('thrush'). It is worth treating the patient for dysbiosis (see box on page 69) to see if this will clear up the toxins and hence the acne. No definitive studies have been done to test whether this link exists, but treatment with the anti-candidal agent, tea tree oil, on acne patients showed there was a good improvement (2).

Where to start?

A nutritional therapist, a herbalist or a homoeopath should be consulted first. The descriptions of treatment may give you a clue as to what could be the cause of your acne and help you make the choice of which route to follow first.

There's a wealth of anecdotal evidence that states acupuncture can help acne but no clinical studies are available to back this up.

DYSBIOSIS

Bacteria exists naturally in our guts to help digest food. Dysbiosis is a disturbance of the normal equilibrium in the growth of these bacteria. It is often accompanied by overgrowth of the fungus, candida. The result of dysbiosis/candidiasis is 'leaky gut'. This means that the walls of the gut allow proteins and carbohydrates to leak out into the bloodstream before they have been broken down to their constituent parts: amino acids and sugars. This results in toxicity as these partly digested chemicals trigger allergic reactions in the body. More discussion of 'leaky gut' is found on page 43 and details of symptoms which may help you decide if you are likely to be suffering from dysbiosis.

NUTRITIONAL THERAPY

This therapy has been found to be successful in the treatment of acne and the following vitamins and mineral supplements are often prescribed to relieve the condition.

Vitamin A: this helps to reduce sebum production. Large doses (up to 50,000 IU daily are needed. The recommended maintenance level is 7500 IU) but this isn't recommended for long periods as vitamin A can be toxic. Strict supervision by an expert is necessary and should only be considered in difficult cases as vitamin A can be a dangerous supplement if overdosed.

Vitamin E & selenium: male acne patients have been shown to have significantly decreased levels of a chemical glutathione peroxidase in their red blood cells. Vitamin E and selenium supplementation inhibits the production of this chemical and improves acne in both men and women (3).

Zinc: this is a potent healer and is lower in 13 and 14 year-old males than any other group (4). It is thought important in the treatment of acne. The majority of patients require at least 12 weeks' supplementation to show any improvement.

HERBAL MEDICINE
Clinical trials have not been carried out to investigate the use of the following herbal remedies but the ones listed have something to offer in the treatment of acne.

● **The saw palm** (*Serenoa repens*) Acne, like prostate overgrowth, is linked to overproduction of dihydrotestosterone. Research has already shown that this plant is useful in the treatment of prostate overgrowth, and so although there isn't as yet any clinical research into its use in acne, it may prove useful, especially in males.

● **Purple coneflower** (*Echinacea angustifolia*) inhibits inflammation, promotes wound healing and stimulates the immune system to kill bacteria.

● **Golden seal** (*Hydrastis canadensis*) has detoxifying and antibacterial properties.

HOMOEOPATHY
Complex homoeopathy is effective in treating acne. (See pages 93–94 for the difference between complex and classical homoeopathy.)

The following classical homoeopathic remedies can help reduce the symptoms of acne (although there are no studies to back this up), but they should be used only if the patient profile and the symptom picture matches the remedy.

Symptom	Remedy
For full-blooded, red-faced people.	Belladonna
For when the pustules are prominent.	Hepar sulph
For pale, fair-haired people.	Pulsatilla
For when there is much scarring.	Silica
For obstinate, long-standing cases.	Sulphur

Eczema

Eczema and dermatitis are itchy inflammations of the skin. These conditions are often hereditary and in recent years eczema in particular has become increasingly common. Both of these conditions share three main symptom patterns, and the skin has some or all of the following appearances.

● Redness and scaling.
● Weeping encrusted sores perhaps with scaling.
● Itching and burning.

Adult eczema usually starts on the face but it can also appear in other places, notably in the folds of the skin – the elbows, knees, buttocks, ankles and wrists. Often the patient has a history of allergic-type diseases in their family such as asthma and hay fever. Eczema is more common in children, although it often clears up before the age of five. It can also develop in later life.

With contact dermatitis, the patient becomes sensitized to a particular allergen with which they are in frequent contact, resulting in skin eruption in the affected area. In many of these cases, contact dermatitis is linked to the patient's occupation. For example, a hairdresser may develop contact dermatitis on his or her hands because of a sensitivity to an ingredient in the shampoo they use daily. A very common sensitivity is to nickel, which is present in many types of jewellery.

Where to start?

Conventional medicine treats contact dermatitis by recommending that you avoid the sensitizer, and steroid creams are generally prescribed to clear up the skin in the case of eczema. These steroids work promptly but long-term use can cause the skin to thin. Complementary medicine treats eczema and dermatitis in a completely different manner, treating the the body as a whole and not just the skin. The underlying cause of the eczema is sought and then treated. Any sensitivity to food, dust or moulds should first be eliminated as a possible cause and desensitization treatment can help with this. A clinical ecologist or a nutritional therapist can help, and the latter can also recommend supplements. If no sensitivity is apparent, herbalism has been shown to be useful, although more research is needed. Acupuncture can also help although treatment may take some months to be effective. Homoeopathy has also proven to be a useful therapy.

CLINICAL ECOLOGY

This treatment can work effectively for eczema, particularly if food sensitivity is involved.

● **Food sensitivity:** this occurs most often to milk and other dairy products, rather than to wheat. Sometimes there is sensitivity to corn (or other cereals) and fruits (especially citrus and tomatoes).

● **Moulds and dust mites:** if the eczema gets worse at night, dust mite allergy should be explored as a cause. You could be reacting to dust mites in the bedding or mattress. Thick curtains and carpets should be avoided, and family pets such as cats and dogs may also be responsible. If the eczema gets worse in winter and damp conditions and improves in hot weather, then mould spores could be triggering it. Densitizing with homoeopathic remedies can help (see Clinical ecology pages 124–130).

NUTRITIONAL MEDICINE

This therapy can help eczema and dermatitis by prescribing supplements such as the following.

● Evening primrose oil is the most common and most successful supplementation and a number of studies have borne this out. High doses are needed: 500mg capsules, three times a day (1).

● It has been shown that some eczema patients are producing too little gastric acid (hydrochloric acid). Giving this as a supplement along with vitamin B has been shown to help in cases which have responded to nothing else (2). Before treatment you should be tested to find out if you are indeed producing insufficient gastric acid. Your doctor can arrange the test.

HERBALISM

Recently, there has been a huge interest in the use of Chinese herbs to treat eczema and there have been definite improvements in some patients. The Royal Free and Great Ormond Street Hospitals in London conducted a trial on 40 adult patients with long-standing eczema and this approach has been proven to work (3). Marigold (*Calendula*) ointment from health food shops can also give skin relief.

ACUPUNCTURE

There are no clinical trials, but there have been good reports of curing eczema with acupuncture. A traditional Chinese approach is best. The acupuncturist determines to what degree there is an imbalance in 'heat', 'damp' and 'wind' and then corrects it. For instance, if the skin is weeping, the 'damp' would be corrected by needling the spleen and stomach points. The liver may also be involved. Treatment can sometimes be lengthy.

HOMOEOPATHY

There have been no clinical trials into the success of homoeopathy with eczema but a number of classical remedies have proven useful:

Symptom	Remedy
For rough, dry skin with cracks.	Graphites
For a pricking rash that is easily infected, is sore to touch and bleeds easily.	Hepar sulph
For eczema that is worse for warmth such as when lying in bed. The eczema is moist.	Mercurius
For itchy, raw, red skin.	Natrum Mur
For skin that is worse for being in a stuffy, hot room, and a hot burning rash that is worse when sweating.	Sulphur

An experienced homoeopath should always be consulted in cases of eczema because, sometimes, following the homoeopathic treatment, the problem can get worse. If this does happens and the condition does not then start to improve, the treatment should be stopped immediately, and sometimes an antidote will be needed.

Psoriasis

Psoriasis is a common skin condition: between two and four people in every 100 have it. It manifests itself in patches of pink covered by silver scaling. It often affects the knees, elbows, trunk, scalp and hairline. Psoriasis is caused by the skin cells reproducing too quickly – at 1,000 times the normal rate. They pile up giving the skin its silvery, scaly appearance.

This arises because of an imbalance in two compounds occurring within cells – cyclic AMP and cyclic GMP – which between them control how the cells multiply and mature. In psoriasis sufferers, something has gone wrong with the interaction between these two compounds and treatment is aimed at restoring the balance so that the cells can grow once more at a normal rate.

Which therapy can help?

Complementary therapy has something to offer with psoriasis, but treatment can be a slow process. It may take some time to isolate what's causing the imbalance. The first person to seek out is probably a nutritional therapist, who can assess if protein digestion is efficient and if the bowel or liver would benefit from detoxifying. The best way to detoxify the liver, if this is necessary, is by homoeopathy and so consulting a homoeopath later in the treatment may also prove to be useful.

Sunlight often clears up psoriasis. Acupuncture has been useful for many patients although there have been no clinical trials to prove this. Usually at least 10 treatments are needed before any significant improvement is seen.

What is causing the imbalance?

There are several possible avenues that should be explored by psoriatic patients to find out the cause.

- Whether protein is being properly digested.
- Whether the bowel would benefit from detoxification.

● Whether the liver is functioning properly.
● Whether alcohol consumption is too high (this affects the liver).
● Whether there is excessive consumption of animal fats (which also affects the liver).

NUTRITIONAL MEDICINE

This therapy is the most highly recommended to help treat psoriasis, and the condition can be looked at from several different areas.

Protein digestion

When protein is digested it is broken down to its 'building blocks' – amino acids. If protein isn't digested properly, or if the resulting amino acids aren't absorbed properly by the body, bacteria breaks down the amino acids into toxins. One group of toxic amino acids are known as polyamines and these have been shown to be increased in patients with psoriasis. Polyamines interfere with the formation of cyclic AMP and therefore speed up the rate of cell growth. Lowering the skin levels of polyamines helps to improve the condition of the psoriasis (1).

Vitamin C, zinc and vitamin A especially inhibit the formation of polyamines and therefore help psoriasis (2).

Toxic bowel

Rosenberg and Belew in 1982 identified that certain toxic compounds which start in the gut due to bacterial action, are implicated in the development of psoriasis. (These include endotoxins [bacteria cell wall fragments], candida and yeast compounds.) These toxins increase cyclic GMP levels within the skin cells and increase the formation of cells (3). Detoxifying the bowel by treating dysbiosis and candida is very important in some cases of psoriasis (see Dysbiosis on page 69).

Psoriatic patients in a Swedish hospital improved on a fasting and vegetarian diet (4), probably because of a decrease in gut-derived toxins and polyamines. Patients have also benefited from a gluten-free diet (5). A nutritional therapist can advise.

Inhibiting the production of irritants which can cause inflammation can be achieved by dosing with 10 to 12g of evening primrose oil according to several well-run clinical studies (6).

Correcting liver function

The liver's job is to detoxify the blood. If the liver is overwhelmed by too many toxins, or if the liver can't filter the toxins properly, the level of these compounds circulating in the blood increases and the psoriasis gets worse (7). Cutting down on alcohol is obviously one means of cutting down on the work the liver has to do.

HOMOEOPATHY

Psoriasis patients also benefit from treatment that strengthens the liver so it can cope better with toxins. The best method of strengthening the liver is with complex homoeopathy and if a malfunctioning liver is suspected, this is a route worth pursuing. (See complex homoeopathy, page 94.)

No clinical trials have been conducted on homoeopathic remedies for psoriasis but the following can prove useful if the patient and symptom profile fits.

Symptom	Remedy
For thick clusters, associated with burning and itching.	Cicuta var
For pustules formed in or under the scaly patches.	Clematix
For when there is thick gummy fluid indicating infection.	Graphites
If warmth makes itching worse and especially if there is lots of scaling.	Kali ars
If there has been much use of paraffin-based ointments.	Petroleum
For when the skin never seems really clean.	Psorinum

2 problems

You may be suffering from a problem which affects your health and general wellbeing but which couldn't exactly be classified as an illness, so what precisely can complementary medicine do to help you in these circumstances?

The answer is quite a lot. Complementary medicine offers good support when you are going through trying circumstances or making difficult lifestyle changes.

Complementary medicine is of no use unless you are determined to eat more healthily and gradually increase the amount of exercise that you take, but once that decision is made, the following complementary therapies will help.

INSOMNIA

Conventional treatment for insomnia (chronic sleeplessness) is usually with strong drugs. Because of the side effects of these drugs, including in some cases, possible addiction, patients usually do not want to be prescribed them for long periods. There are several complementary options to try. The herb valerian is probably a good place to start because it seems to be as useful as drugs in helping sleeplessness, but experimenting with the amount of caffeine and alcohol consumed at the same time is advisable. If this fails, it is worth consulting a nutritional therapist about possible tryptophan supplementation.

● Valerian is a well-known sedative and recent trials have shown that it can relieve insomnia and help improve the quality of sleep.

In one trial 44 per cent of insomniacs reported perfect sleep and 89 per cent improved sleep. There were no side effects or 'hangover' feelings the next morning as you would expect with drugs (1).

● Drinking a little alcohol may help. Drinking a lot of alcohol could disturb sleep more. At low doses of alcohol, sleeping time is increased but, it should be noted that even a little alcohol reduces the amount of REM sleep (rapid eye movement – the best sleep for alleviating tiredness the next day). It is probably down to the individual to experiment with different levels of alcohol consumption – including abstention – to see what works best (2).

● Caffeine is also linked to insomnia. A group of 4,558 Australians reported increased wakefulness with higher caffeine intake (3). There is caffeine in tea and also in fizzy drinks, such as cola as well as coffee.

● The natural chemical tryptophan, is converted into serotonin, which is important for inducing and maintaining sleep. It has been found that 1g of tryptophan before going to bed causes people to fall asleep more quickly. For people with mild or moderate insomnia dosage at around this level may help. It is of most use to patients with low levels of sleeplessness. Chronic insomniacs do not respond as well at first but if they carry on with the treatment, their sleep patterns improve, implying that the tryptophan has a cumulative effect. They may however need a higher dose. Too high a dose can actually cause sleep disturbance but taking around 10 to 15 mg is considered safe (4).

GIVING UP SMOKING

This is the single most important choice that people can make to protect their health. However, although help is available in giving up smoking, it has to be realized that there is no 'magic' cure. You have to want to give up. Nothing will help unless the smoker is serious about wanting to stop.

How does complementary medicine fare when set against orthodox medicine's answer, nicotine replacement? According to research, fairly well. Acupuncture and hypnosis both have achieved results as good as nicotine replacement when it comes to quitting (about 15 per cent of patients were still not smoking after 6 months). From the point of view of effectiveness, the success rates are roughly comparable. Both have been known to work well with patients who have tried other methods and failed.

From the point of view of cost, there is a case for trying hypnotherapy first. In some studies, patients have needed only one or two sessions, with acupuncture two to four sessions (as with most acupuncture treatments) are needed. But if one doesn't work, and you are still quite convinced that you want to stop, try the other method which might suit you better.

Acupuncture

When an overview of seven studies into giving up smoking and acupuncture was made (over 500 patients were involved), acupuncture's success rate at six months after the treatment was about 25 per cent (1). What's interesting is that it didn't really seem to matter where the needles were inserted, which has led doctors to think that acupuncture helps in stopping smoking by triggering the release of endorphins (chemicals which promote feelings of wellbeing in the body) (2). Acupuncture is at least as effective as nicotine replacement therapy.

Several different acupuncture methods are used, but often a small, semi-permanent needle is placed in the ear. When the individual wants to smoke, they twiddle with this needle instead, causing endorphins to be released in the body which dampen down the withdrawal symptoms and lessen the need for a cigarette.

A couple of sessions are needed, perhaps as many as four. If the smoker has not stopped or cut down substantially after four sessions, acupuncture is not likely to help. But remember that this doesn't mean acupuncture won't help in the future, when the smoker's frame of mind towards smoking may change or become more positive.

Hypnotherapy

It's been said that hypnotherapy is a brilliantly effective way of helping people to achieve what they already want to do (3), and this is never truer than when it comes to giving up smoking.

If you are considering hypnotherapy, it is important to understand that the therapy is just a tool and you have to take responsibility for its success or failure. If you carry on smoking, it is your fault, not the therapy's; but if you do stop smoking, the credit is all yours. Unlike acupuncture, hypnotherapy does not provide any biochemical support, but it does reinforce your own decision to quit.

Certainly, if you are committed, you will have already have thought carefully about it and decided the reasons why you want to give up; hypnosis will put you in a receptive state where you will be more open to these ideas.

What's actually suggested to you by the hypnotherapist during the trance state varies: several approaches are used. The smoker will already want to quit for health reasons and the positive aspects of giving up can be reinforced during the trance. While in this highly susceptible state, building up a loathing of cigarettes (aversion) by focusing on how disgusting cigarettes smell and taste is another approach. Telling patients that the addiction is not difficult to give up and building the expectation that they won't desire a cigarette after the session has also worked well.

The *Practitioner* reported in 1985 that in a study of 683 patients a single session of hypnotherapy helped between 30 to 40 per cent of patients to give up smoking a year later (4).

Self hypnosis is also a possible method. In one study, patients were given counselling and then taught how to hypnotize themselves with the instruction to do it three to 10 times a day (as needed). Out of 616 patients, 35 per cent were cigarette-free a year later (5).

Tapes are available to help with self-hypnosis and this may seem attractive, but the counselling part of the above treatment was probably important. The attention of a therapist seems to be an important ingredient in the therapeutic mix.

This is borne out by examining the success rates of hypnotherapy in several other studies. Several researchers have reported that between 12 and 25 per cent of patients quit following a single session of hypnotherapy, but in another study when counselling was added to a single hypnosis session the quit rate rose to 53 per cent (6).

There is also evidence that hypnotherapy works best when used with other mind–body therapies. In the most successful results yet for hypnotherapy, 88 per cent of a group of 60 smokers were still smoke-free one year after a 15 minute session of individual hypnotism coupled with some group learning of relaxation, imagery and self-hypnosis techniques (7).

It's a good idea to find a therapist who has had a lot of experience in helping people give up smoking. A single treatment can be helpful (see above) but booking in for a few sessions will increase your chances of giving up completely.

STRESS

Stress is commonly talked about today. Just about any condition is attributed at least in part to stress and it is seen as the universal evil. But the truth is that a little stress is good for us, it motivates and inspires us. But when we are overburdened by problems that we just cannot solve on a daily basis, that is when stress becomes a problem and we are in danger of getting ill.

All of the following conditions or symptoms can be caused by stress: allergies; anxiety and depression; digestive and bowel problems; skin disorders; heart disease; migraines and headaches; insomnia; and menstrual problems.

Solutions to these various conditions can be found elsewhere in this book, but if you know that you have a very stressful lifestyle and that it is the major cause of your symptom(s), then dealing with it will go a long way to help resolve your problem.

Many of the complementary therapies detailed in this book can help stress-related problems as they are aimed at restoring balance to the body system, but the following therapies can act quickly to calm you.

● First, consider taking up one of the mind–body therapies such as yoga or meditation (see pages 130–140). This is one of the fastest routes to dealing with stress on a deep level. But they still take time, the very thing that many stressed people feel they haven't got. Unfortunately, short of adopting a completely different career or lifestyle, the only cure for stress is devoting some time on a daily basis to attending to your own needs. If practising a mind–body therapy on a regular basis seems too much, or if you are feeling depressed or in some other way unable to cope with one right now, at least put aside one hour a week for massage, reflexology or a healing session. The act of 'giving' yourself this hour a week to focus on yourself and your needs is often the start towards a more balanced lifestyle.

● Your diet should be looked at carefully. Many people who are exhausted simply don't eat enough good-quality food, including plenty of fresh fruit and vegetables, at regular intervals to ensure that their body has a steady flow of energy. Women especially tend to suffer from a deficiency in the B vitamins and magnesium which are both important for maintaining a healthy nervous system. Stress depletes reserves of vitamins and minerals even faster. A nutritional therapist can advise if a mineral or vitamin supplement might benefit you.

● Alcohol, caffeine and cigarettes are the 'friends' we turn to in an attempt to calm us down when we are stressed. As we all know these actually make symptoms of stress worse, and although giving them up or cutting them down in the short-term is stressful in itself, you will very quickly feel the benefits.

● A good acupuncturist can help to rebalance a stressed system, and strengthen your body to cope with the demands placed on it during stressful times.

3 therapies

ACUPUNCTURE

Acupuncture is used to diagnose illness and promote future health by stimulating the body's self-healing powers. This is achieved by 'triggering' certain points on the body with needles. Research has shown that acupuncture alters a person's perception of pain, increases their immune response, normalizes their body's functions and also has a tranquillizing effect.

Probably, the first question in your mind about acupuncture is not so much 'does it work?' but 'does it hurt?' The fact that you can heal disease by inserting needles into the surface of the skin, in what seems a haphazard arrangement, is a hard one for the Western mind to accept, especially if you are not too keen on needles.

So first, it should be pointed out that the needles used penetrate only very superficially and that the needles themselves are tiny – think of the dimensions of a single hair. The experience is far less traumatic than having an injection (where the needles are designed to pass through the skin). Acupuncture can have a profound effect on your body, but it should not prove to be a painful experience.

It is a very ancient therapy; archaeologists have found stone needles that date back to 3,000 BC. The Egyptians also used a form of acupuncture, but it is the Chinese who refined it into a system of medicine. The first Chinese medical text book was a book on acupuncture. *Huang Di Nei Jing (The Yellow Emperor's Classic of Internal Medicine)* which dates back to 475-221 BC.

Over the centuries, acupuncture travelled westwards and was fairly popular in the later half of the eighteenth century but it fell into disrepute by the nineteenth century. Even in China, there was an attempt to ban it following the overthrow of the imperial family in 1911. Many practitioners and teachers were persecuted during the Cultural Revolution but Traditional Chinese Medicine and acupuncture survived.

In an attempt to improve relations that were destroyed during the Cultural Revolution, the Chinese Government invited the American president, Richard Nixon for a state visit in 1972. At that time, acupuncture was brought to the notice of the American physicians that he had with him, and fuelled by their positive reaction a wave of fresh interest in acupuncture spread through the West.

How does it work?

THE CHINESE VIEW

Much of traditional Chinese medicine is based on Taoist thought – a philosophical system which teaches that for harmony to exist there must be a fundamental balance to the world.

Chi

As with everything, the body's natural state also needs to be balanced. There are two forces, yin (dark, passive and feminine) and yang (light, active and male) which are both opposite and interdependent. True health – emotional and physical – is only possible when yin and yang are in balance. According to the Chinese tradition, there are six main organs which are yin and six which are yang. Each yin organ is linked structurally to its yang organ. A breakdown in one organ will have a 'knock on' effect on other parts of the body. The organs are also related to emotions. A disruption of the body's natural harmony thus manifests itself in both physical and emotional problems.

According to Chinese tradition, when yin and yang are not in balance, Chi cannot flow smoothly through out bodies and when Chi is blocked, stagnant or weakened, illness arises. There is no clear Western definition of Chi. Think of it as your 'vital energy' or 'life force' which drives each and every cell. Modern research has described it in terms of electromagnetic energy.

The Chinese believe that this energy flows through your body in 12 channels or 'meridians' – six are yin and six are yang – and eight deeper channels. Along these meridians are specific points which can be stimulated by needles and result in a greater flow of Chi. In Traditional Chinese Medicine there are more than 800 points. Chi is vital to the body as it supports, nourishes and protects your emotional, physical and mental wellbeing.

Normally there is a state of relative harmony within the body and between the body and the environment. But both our internal and our external environments are constantly changing, and whether or not we succumb to disease depends on how well we adapt to these changes. These include external stressors such as the weather or bacteria and internal ones like the shock of a bereavement or the emotion of self-pity. This leads to a deficiency or excess of Chi in one or more parts of the body (see box below) which will affect the whole system. If such an imbalance does occur, acupuncture can rebalance the flow of Chi by stimulating the relevant points on the body. Where appropriate, herbs and dietary modifications may be prescribed as well to help restore harmony more quickly.

TAOISM

Taoism also teaches that the emotions affect the body.
Each organ is linked to an emotion.

- **Joy**   **heart/small intestine**
- **Obsession, worry**   **spleen/stomach**
- **Sadness, grief**   **lungs/large intestine**
- **Fear, fright**   **kidney/bladder**
- **Anger**   **liver/gallbladder**

THE WESTERN VIEW

Faced with indisputable, visible proof that acupuncture worked, especially at relieving pain, it's hardly surprising that Western scientists were intrigued, and attempted to find an explanation which fits in with our theories of human physiology.

The one that most clearly seems to explain acupuncture's effects is that it causes the release of key chemicals (neurotransmitters) which carry messages between nerve endings. The release of these neurotransmitters blocks the sensation of pain. (This theory is given credence by the fact that a functioning nervous system is necessary for acupuncture to work; if the nerves are cut to an area, acupuncture will not produce an analgesic [painkilling] effect.)

The release of these neurotransmitters may also explain other physiological changes which acupuncture is known to achieve: for instance, acupuncture can have an anti-inflammatory effect and alleviate the pain of inflamed joints, by releasing two natural anti-inflammatory chemicals. Acupuncture can also significantly reduce a raised blood pressure, and this too may be due to the release of neurotransmitters which in turn trigger the release of hormones which act on the blood vessels.

But not all the effects of acupuncture can be explained by Western science. Until we discover more about the workings of the human body, much is still a mystery.

Which ailments can it help?

Acupuncture works particularly well as a preventative treatment and on the ailment front The World Health Organization drew up a list in 1979 of 104 ailments which acupuncture had been reported to help. This was based largely on Chinese reports and not all of it would be sufficient evidence for Western clinical trials. However, in the experience of practitioners at The Centre for the Study of Complementary Medicine at Southampton the following conditions have been helped by acupuncture.

● **Painful disorders** such as headaches, migraine, osteoarthritis, back pain, sciatica, frozen shoulder and sports' injuries. Acupuncture has been estimated to give relief from chronic pain in 55 to 80 per cent of cases compared to 70 per cent with morphine and 30 to 35 per cent with placebo.

● **Respiratory disorders** such as sinusitis, asthma and bronchitis.

● **Cardiovascular disorders** such as high blood pressure and illnesses where the blood flow to parts of the body is diminished.

● **Gut disorders** such as irritable bowel syndrome, inflammatory bowel disease, gastritis and colic.

- **Gynaecological disorders** such as painful periods and PMS.
- **Skin disorders** such as eczema, psoriasis, acne and hives.
- **Anxiety, depression** and **insomnia**.
- **Allergies** such as food sensitivity.
- **Addictions** such as smoking, excess drinking and overeating.

What can you expect?

On your first appointment, your acupuncturist will take a very detailed case history: you will be asked about your general health, that of your parents and other close relatives; your eating habits, work schedule and sleeping pattern. Your tongue will be examined carefully and the acupuncturist will take your pulse. This is a more complex process than when your doctor does it. Each wrist is measured in turn but instead of feeling for one pulse, the acupuncturist is feeling for six on each wrist. By checking your pulses the acupuncturist is assessing how well your Chi is flowing and pinpointing blockages or weaknesses and this can take several minutes. The pulse taking may be repeated throughout the session after the needles have been inserted in order to assess how well the treatment is working.

You will be asked to lie on a couch, most probably on your back. Since the acupuncturist will need access to points all over your body, you will probably be asked to remove your outer clothes and wear only underwear for the actual treatment.

Once the needles are inserted in the relevant points, you will be left alone to lie quietly while the needles do their work, possibly listening to relaxing music. A period of about 20 minutes is usually considered ideal to allow the flow of Chi to correct itself. After this time, the acupuncturist will examine your pulses again and make notes of his or her findings.

Acupuncture should not hurt. For the most part, a pinprick as you are 'needled' is all you should feel. Sometimes a heavy, dull ache or a warm sensation is felt due to Chi flowing to that point. The perception of pain however is subjective. Occasionally, there may be a little blood as if from a pinprick, but this is rare; sometimes there is some very minor bruising. Normally, there is no sign of where the needles have been inserted. Therapists report that a small number of patients experience more discomfort than others and over-tense patients may fall into this category. Usually an acupuncturist will insert around eight needles in any one session, although it can be less.

Sometimes, there will be a short, sharp pain as one particular point is 'needled' – this is a sign that the point is related to a strong blockage. For instance, a patient suffering from a bad cold may experience a slight pain when a needle is inserted in a point related to phlegm; another person who is 'broken-hearted' at the end of an affair, may feel a sharper sensation when the therapist treats a 'heart' point. This should not put you off; the pain lasts a second and is a clear sign that your therapist knows what she is doing.

You may feel euphoric or revitalized after acupuncture. You will almost certainly feel relaxed which is why it's a good idea to make sure you don't have anything too strenuous to cope with after your appointment. Ideally, you should relax afterwards to allow the change in the flow of Chi to take place.

Certain factors can affect the flow of Chi – the diagnosis, and the treatment itself – and you should particularly try to avoid the following activities or emotions before or after treatment as they can cause dizziness.

- Alcohol.
- Heavy meals.
- Missing meals and feeling hungry.
- Sex.
- Hot baths.
- Being emotional upset.
- Being excessively tired.

OTHER ACUPUNCTURE TREATMENTS

Moxibustion The moxa herb is burnt at the end of the needles on the points that need further stimulation. The patient doesn't experience burning but needs to tell the practitioner when it feels hot. The heat works to promote the flow of Chi.

Electroacupuncture A pulsed electric current is used to stimulate acupuncture needles. This stimulus is thought to increase the efficacy of 'needling' and is particularly popular with doctors who are trained in Western medicine but also practise acupuncture.

Laser acupuncture Low-level lasers are used to stimulate traditional points. The process is completely painless and doesn't involve needles but uses pen-like tools which give out an infrared low-power beam, so it is likely to appeal to children or those with a phobia about needles. However, this is still in its infancy and it is not yet clear if it is as effective as using needles.

Cupping This is used all the time in China but less often here as it can sometimes cause bruising which might prove unacceptable to Western patients. Glass, metal, wood or bamboo cups are heated and then placed over specific points to bring Chi quickly to that area.

How long does treatment take?

An acute (short-term) condition will respond fairly quickly to treatment. A chronic (long-term) condition will take longer. Most acupuncturists expect to see a definite improvement in an ailment after about four to six treatments and often suggest at the initial consultation that there is a review of progress after six treatments where you can both assess whether you think it worth carrying on.

For advice on how to find an acupuncturist see page 148.

THE PRACTITIONER
Gerry Harris is a practising acupuncturist.

'I'm an impatient person and what drew me to practise acupuncture, rather than another therapy, was that in minutes you can tell, from the pulses, whether you've achieved something. If you don't get a pulse change, you haven't done a treatment.

'It can give quick relief for painful conditions and it can help patients on an emotional level because as the balance is restored, you are given the chance to choose how to behave. So if you're an angry person, who steams into a situation and thinks afterwards, you will find yourself less likely to do that. You'll find yourself standing back and deciding if you want to steam in or not.'

THE DOCTOR/PRACTITIONER
Dr Fiona Bolden uses acupuncture within her general practice.

'From the very beginning I'd always thought that Western medicine was a bit limited. I went to New Zealand to work for a while and got interested in the idea of treating people 'energetically' (treating their energy), but I didn't know how to do it. I discovered acupuncture and studied it for three years while still working as a doctor in Britain. Then I went to China and saw that acupuncture could be used alongside Western medicine.

'My patients were very amenable and open-minded about trying acupuncture and so far it has worked very well. Far more people approach me about it than I can possibly treat. However, I'm quite careful to work only on the patients who I believe will benefit so my success rate is high.'

CASE HISTORY
Freddie, a trader, has osteoarthritis in both knees, his spine, hands and ankles and turned to acupuncture for some pain relief.

'I have a fruit and veg stall at our local market – it's hard physical work and you're outside in all weathers – which isn't very helpful for the arthritis. My arthritis got gradually worse over 10 years and I was on anti-inflammatory drugs for six years. Although they took the pain away there were unpleasant side effects such as stomach upsets. When my doctor told me she was going to do blood tests to see if the drugs had damaged my liver and kidneys, I started thinking, this is ridiculous, I can't take something every day that's poisoning me – there must be another way of managing this without using drugs.

'I read everything I could and started doing the Hay food combining diet. It sounds complicated but after a while it's as easy as anything. I also gave up alcohol and red meat and started meditating. I was then offered the chance to have acupuncture but I hate needles. I've even fainted before having an injection. I was so nervous the first time I went I thought I was going to freak out and run up the street. I've now had five treatments and I still don't like it. I shut my eyes and try to put myself in another place while the needles are inserted. But it's worth it because it works for me. After the first treatment I was wiped out, and more tired than I've ever been in my life. After the second treatment I thought I was cured. I felt I'd been let out of prison – the pain had gone away. But it did come back. What I'm finding is that I'm pain-free for longer periods after each treatment. I've gone three full days without experiencing any pain and my wife noticed something the other day – I ran up the stairs. Before that I had been walking with a stick to stop me falling over. I've got some hope now that eventually I will be free from pain. I used to be a guitar player but I couldn't play because a joint in my hand was affected. Now I'm telling myself, "see how you get on, you might be playing the guitar again one day" '.

CASE HISTORY
Darren, an import and stock clerk, has suffered from back problems for years.

'My back problems first started when I helped someone push their car out of a ditch. My back went. It was so painful I couldn't get into work. Apparently I displaced something and it's gone three times since. It usually takes two to three weeks to settle down. I've tried osteopathy which has helped somewhat to speed up recovery.

'The last time my back went, I'd been stripping wallpaper from the ceiling and the strain affected my neck. I couldn't turn it. I took painkillers and rested and used hot water bottles for seven days, but my neck actually got worse. I went to the hospital after a week and the only thing I didn't want was a neck collar because I'd been told they make things worse. The doctor didn't offer me that but she asked how I felt about trying acupuncture – I agreed to try it as I was up for anything.

'The doctor, as it happened, was one who practised acupuncture. She stuck two needles into my neck. I didn't feel anything at first, but just 20 to 30 minutes later it had loosened up and about five hours later I could move my neck as much as I wanted. I was quite impressed. Osteopathy was good but it didn't work as quickly as acupuncture. My back will always be my weak point and I'm pleased I've now got acupuncture to help relieve the pain.'

HOMOEOPATHY

We owe our knowledge of homoeopathy as we know it today to a German physician Samuel Hahnemann, although the Greek physician Hippocrates was known to have used homoeopathic remedies back in 430 BC. Hahnemann was a visionary in the late 1700s who was so disgusted by the cruel, and to his mind, fairly useless medical treatments of his time (leaching, purging and using poison), that he gave up practising medicine and devoted his energies to research and translating medical papers. While translating a book by a Scot, one Dr William Cullen, Hahnemann's curiosity was aroused by Cullen's statement that quinine cured malaria because of its 'bitter' qualities.

Hahnemann doubted these findings but began his own investigations into quinine's actions by dosing himself with it. To his amazement, he went on to develop malaria-like symptoms. He tested quinine on other people and the pattern was repeated. He also discovered that the severity of the symptoms depended on the individual and concluded that the person's own healing capacity played a part in their reaction to the drug. From these observations developed what are still two fundamental tenets of homoeopathy: that 'like cures like' and that since each individual's response to treatment is different, the cure must be tailored specifically to that individual.

Traditional Western medicine is a form of 'allopathic' medicine. 'Allo-' is derived from the Greek for 'other'. So if you have a bad cold your doctor will give you treatment to oppose and suppress your symptoms – an antipyretic to bring down fever, an antibiotic to kill the bug causing it. This is the opposite approach to that of the homoeopath who will see your fever and blocked nose as the body's struggle to heal itself. Homoeopathy is derived from the Greek word 'homios' for 'similar'. The homoeopath's remedy is aimed at supporting the body's own efforts. You are treated with a remedy which in larger doses would bring on the very symptoms you're trying to shake off.

Classical homoeopathic remedies are prepared by taking either a plant or mineral source and macerating it in alcohol and water. This is then strained and the result is called the 'mother tincture'. The mother tincture is then dissolved with water, sometimes many hundreds of times, to form the remedy which is given to patients. The dilution process is often carried out to such an extent that it has been estimated that not one molecule of the original mother tincture could remain. It is one of the paradoxes of this medical system that homoeopaths have found that the very dilute remedies are more beneficial than higher concentrations.

Since Hahnemann's time all the greatest homoeopaths have been American, and in the United States and in other European countries, another kind of homoeopathy, known as 'complex homoeopathy' has arisen, which differs slightly from the 'classical' approach described above. This type of homoeopathy uses herbs and sometimes extracts from animal organs in conjunction with the remedies. The complex homoeopathic cures using organ material are particularly beneficial to the equivalent organ in the human patient. Whereas classical homoeopathy works on a very subtle level to treat the whole body, complex homoeopathy remedies are aimed at alleviating a particular symptom and often work directly on one organ of the body. Complex homoeopathy does not depend so much on matching the patient to the remedy and is used a lot by doctors who practise homoeopathy. The results are often a bit quicker than with classical homoeopathy.

How does it work?

Quite how homoeopathy works is unknown. Hahnemann believed in what he called 'vital force' which is the natural healing energy in our bodies, and which is stimulated by homoeopathic remedies. He could not explain scientifically how they worked, but he showed that they did from the success of his treatments.

Common sense tells us that it simply shouldn't work – it goes against the basis of Western scientific reasoning. How can, what is basically water, have any therapeutic benefit, say the sceptics?

But homoeopathy does work. It just does not work in any way which can be explained by straightforward biochemistry. We will have to wait for new ideas to explain it fully, but these ideas are beginning to come through. The 'chaos' theory – the one which teaches that tiny movements such as the flap of a butterfly's wing can set in motion colossal events like a typhoon – may prove to be applicable to the effects of homoeopathy. Another route of research is the emerging evidence that water may have some sort of 'memory' imprint (1).

Which ailments can it help?

Five different people who visit their doctor complaining of joint pain will probably be prescribed the same drug, but five visiting a homoeopath will almost certainly leave with different prescriptions. Homoeopathy has been found to help many ailments, but it does not work for everyone and because of the emphasis on the individual, homoeopathy is difficult to assess by clinical trial.

However, an overview of clinical studies into homoeopathy appeared in the British Medical Journal in 1991. It concluded that there was sufficient evidence from well-run clinical trials to prove that homoeopathy did work for the following conditions.

- **Asthma, hay fever** and **upper respiratory tract infections.**
- **Irritable bowel syndrome** and other gut disorders.
- **Skin conditions.**
- **Mental** and **psychological disorders**, for example, insomnia, depression and behavioural problems in children.
- **High blood pressure.**
- **Migraine.**

What can you expect?

A homoeopath will take an exhaustive case history on your first visit. He or she will not only be interested in your present symptoms and previous medical history but will ask seemingly bewildering questions: are you scared of the dark, which is your favourite season, do you like sweet and sour food? The point is to build up a 'picture' of you – of your emotional, physical, mental and spiritual state – which is just as important in prescribing a treatment as the symptoms which have taken you there in the first place. The homoeopath is not treating your symptoms, he or she is treating you, and the skill in homoeopathy is in matching you with one of any number of remedies which could cause your symptoms.

How long does treatment take?

Depending on your illness, and whether the prescription needs to be altered, your homoeopath may ask to see you anything between a week or a month after your initial consultation. It can take around three to four months to see improvement for a chronic (long-term) illness. However, homoeopathy should act fairly swiftly in acute (short-term) conditions – improvement should be noticed within two to four weeks. In cases of a cold, for instance, you should see improvement in hours or days. If you see no improvement after four sessions, it may be worth consulting another homoeopath or trying another therapy.

For advice on how to find a qualified homoeopath see pages 150–151.

THE PRACTITIONER
Dr Tessa Katz is a practising hospital doctor and homoeopath.

'As a doctor, I felt I needed extra tools. It was so frustrating just handing out antibiotics to patients to cure their complaints – I wanted a kind of medicine that is more respectful to the patient and now I use both orthodox and complementary medicine. I was first impressed by seeing how successfully rheumatoid patients were treated with homoeopathy. If it was caught early enough it stopped the disease process. Now practising medicine has become much more challenging and inspiring.'

THE PRACTITIONER
Dr Martin Twine is a GP who uses homoeopathy in his practice.

'Homoeopathy allows maximum improvement in a patient. The healing systems are harnessed instead of being forced by chemical drugs. I have used it successfully for depression, recurrent headaches, anxiety and bad period pain. It isn't a cure for cancer but then it does bring comfort to those who are suffering from terminal disease.'

CASE HISTORY
Anne, a teacher, was knocked flat by an unidentifiable virus.

'I suddenly started feeling very unwell and I had to take to my bed for a couple of weeks. I was tired but the main symptoms were strange tingling sensations in my muscles accompanied by hot and cold attacks. Standing up was impossible. It could have been flu but my doctor wouldn't commit himself to a diagnosis.

'After two weeks I could get up. I took some time off to recover but then had to go back to work. I was a great deal better but then I got quite ill again, and the tingling sensations remained. My doctor couldn't do any more for me because I was getting better but I wanted to get back to full strength quickly. Both my parents have complementary therapy treatments and it helps them. I had always thought it was a bit cranky, but I remember saying to my doctor, "It can't do me any harm and it can only help".

'I was given two homoeopathic treatments – one to detoxify me and one to build up my immune system. After taking them for a few days I got worse, and my back got very stiff. I wasn't too worried as it said on the bottle that things might get worse for a while, but I did stop taking the treatment for a couple of days on the advice of the homoeopath.
'Very gradually, over the course of two months, I did get better. Of course, I'm not sure how much of it would have happened anyway but I know that the treatment was having some definite effect – my body started making some very anti-social noises thanks to the detoxifiying treatment! I did trust my practitioner and that makes a difference. I'm sure, just like anything else, some aren't terribly good. And I'm certainly open to trying it again. I think when you're

reasonably healthy, there isn't much more your doctor can do for you, but homoeopathy treats your whole being and can get you fighting fit faster.'

CASE HISTORY
Laura, a schoolgirl, has suffered from asthma since she was a child.

'I'm 14 now, and I've had asthma since I was six or seven. I've always relied on inhalers and in the morning I was very wheezy. Sports were difficult to play and I often got very congested. My mum was already having homoeopathic treatment and she wanted me to try it, too.

'I'm allergic to pollen, dust mites, moulds and dairy products. The pills I was given helped to reduce my allergic reaction to these things. I took them for about two years, but I started feeling better after a couple of months.

'Two months ago, my doctor took me off the inhaler, although I still have it around in case it's needed. But I haven't had to use it in that time, and I'm no longer on the homoeopathic pills either. My asthma's now under control and I'm absolutely sure it was the homoeopathy that did it – it couldn't have been anything else. I think it's brilliant.'

MANIPULATIVE THERAPIES
(Osteopathy and Chiropractic)

Manipulative therapies are literally 'hands-on' therapies. Physiotherapy is also a type of manipulative treatment but here we're looking at the so-called 'alternatives' – osteopathy and chiropractic. Actually they are less alternative than any of the other treatments discussed in this book. Osteopathy is now much more accepted in Great Britain and patients are often referred for treatment by their doctors. In the United States, chiropractors are medically qualified.

Osteopaths have been canvassing for some time to be given the same kind of credibility by the medical profession that physiotherapists enjoy. And they have now won the struggle (see page 151). There are few doctors who would not consider osteopathy as an extremely valuable treatment. The image of osteopaths and chiropractors as 'bone crushers' has disappeared during the last two decades.

How does it work?

Osteopathy works on the principle that 'structure governs function'. In other words, if the body is misaligned or carries tension (the 'structure'), then a strain is put on the whole body, leading to a malfunctioning system and poor health (the 'function'). This tension or misalignment can be due to any number of things, including poor posture, injury and negative emotions. Relieving the tension or misalignment allows the body to run like a well-oiled machine. The therapists also teach that the mind and body are linked, and the body is treated as a whole. Tension which accumulates in the musculoskeletal system invariably will affect our emotions and mood. Relaxing your muscles allows the circulation, excretory organs and hormonal system to work more efficiently.

Many of the above principles apply to chiropractic. However, osteopaths work on the whole body whereas chiropractors concentrate on the spine. The reason for the emphasis on the spine is that the nerves which serve the entire body run through it. Chiropractors believe that a healthy spine is fundamental to good health, and that much ill health is caused by misalignments of the spinal vertebrae, pressing on nerves and tissues nearby and therefore affecting distant parts of the body.

Chiropractors work on treating one vertebral joint at a time. They often use X-rays to help determine spinal 'subluxations' (you will have to pay for these separately). A subluxation occurs when there is a misalignment of a spinal vertebra so that it is less mobile and this in turn affects the nerves and tissues around it.

SHOULD YOU CONSULT
A CHIROPRACTOR OR OSTEOPATH ?

Because they are so similar, it is difficult to say. The section on 'which ailments can it can help?' may give you some clues as to what will work best for your condition. However, the major differences between the disciplines are listed below.

● Chiropractors concentrate on the spine and always use spinal manipulation; osteopaths also work on the spine, but tend to work over the whole body, using techniques such as massage as well as manipulation.

● Chiropractors often use X-rays for diagnosis and osteopaths rarely do. (If you are pregnant, a chiropractor would not use an X-ray.)

● Some people don't like the 'clicking' sound of the adjustments which are a fundamental part of chiropractic. Osteopathy can be carried out without these adjustments, though, so it might suit some people better. It depends more on massage and traction.

Which ailments can it help?

Osteopathy and chiropractic work especially well for all musculoskeletal problems: bad back, neck pain, frozen shoulder, sciatica, the back pain caused by pregnancy and sports' injuries. Migraine can be treated if the pain is related to tension. Gut problems such as indigestion, constipation and breathing problems, such as asthma, can also be helped. There have been cases of chiropractic restoring hearing loss, and dizziness associated with inner ear imbalances can be helped by both treatments. Immobility because of an arthritic condition can also be helped but osteopathy isn't advisable if the joints are inflamed.

Osteopathy and chiropractic should be avoided with certain medical conditions, these include patients with bone cancer and broken bones. Osteopathy is not advised in patients with osteoporosis (bone thinning) and inflamed joints, although these patients may be able to have chiropractic treatment.

What can you expect?

The first consultation takes about an hour. The osteopath will want to know what type of problem you are experiencing. If you are in pain, he will want to know what kind of pain you have – where it is, what it feels like, how long you've had it. A thorough case history will be taken, including details of previous illnesses, your lifestyle (hobbies, exercise habits, sports), as well as your sleep pattern. Osteopaths check your height and weight. Chiropractors sometimes take blood pressure and pulse. You may also be asked about allergies and diet.

Then the therapist will want to conduct a physical examination. For this, it is usual to strip down to your underwear. You will be asked to walk, sit, bend. All of this is so that the practitioner can see how your body works and check for any misalignments. You may be asked to resist pressure applied to certain joints (although obviously nothing that would cause you pain).

Chiropractors may also take X-rays to confirm the position of subluxations. The actual treatment may not start until the next session when the results of the X-rays are available.

The therapist will tell you what she thinks is wrong and whether or not she can help you. If the answer is 'yes', she will probably relax the muscles by massaging or applying heat treatments before manipulation begins.

Manipulation at the worst should be no more than slightly uncomfortable. Many of the techniques used are gentle. Some like the 'high velocity thrust' are more forceful. The high velocity thrust is a method of realigning the joint. You will be asked to breathe in and the therapist will very quickly apply pressure into a joint. It isn't painful, but it does release gas trapped in the fluid around the joint and can cause a sharp 'crack'. That crack is often the most frightening part of the treatment. Patients understandably think it is the bone that is cracking, but it is only the gas bubbles bursting in the joint. The thrust takes no more than a couple of seconds.

When the manipulation is over, the therapist may give you some exercises to practice and general tips on posture and altering your lifestyle to help your body to recover. She may also advise you on diet or nutritional supplementation if appropriate

After treatment, some people feel terrific, especially if pain has been lifted. Others feel sleepy. Often you feel a bit sore for the next couple of days and as has been pointed out previously, you may, rarely, feel worse. This should always be reported to your practitioner.

How long does treatment take?

Manipulative therapies often have instant results. The pain experienced can disappear after one session, although pain relief may only be temporary and more treatments may be needed.

If you don't feel any better after one treatment, it is still worth having another. But if after three or four treatments, you are still no better then perhaps manipulation is not the solution for you.

In the unlikely case that the pain gets worse (which sometimes happens as part of the healing process), you should report it to the osteopath or chiropractor right away. The original diagnosis may have been wrong, and they may want to reconsider their treatment plan or refer you to someone else.

Most chronic (long-term) conditions are sorted out after about six or seven treatments and it is worth continuing for as long as you can see improvement.

WHAT IS A McTIMONEY CHIROPRACTOR?

A McTimoney chiropractor can treat you as well as any other chiropractor. The main difference is that the treatment is very gentle and that McTimoney chiropractors don't concentrate solely on the spine, they work over the whole body, which some people may find preferable. They also do not rely on X-rays as much. McTimoney chiropractors can help with all the problems that chiropractors treat.

WHAT IS CRANIAL OSTEOPATHY?

Cranial osteopathy is a very gentle technique where the practitioner manipulates the bones of the skull to adjust any imbalances in the cerebrospinal fluid that flows down through the skull to the spine. This treatment can particularly help children who have traumatic births; it can also help adults who are suffering from migraines, dizziness and sinus problems.

For advice on how to find a qualified osteopath or chiropractor see pages 151–152.

THE PRACTITIONER
Fiona Walsh is a practising osteopath

'My job allows me to help people on all sorts of different levels. I have the time to do this and I feel I can really get to grips with the effects that the stress and strain of daily life puts on my patients' health. I have plenty of time to help patients understand what they can do to help themselves, whereas doctors often have to rely on stop-gap measures which treat only the surface of the problem because the patients are in and out so quickly.'

CASE HISTORY
On returning from a trip abroad, Ros, a marketing executive, was incapacitated by severe shoulder pain.

'I had just got back from a business trip abroad, where I had traipsed all over the United States carrying my suitcases. On my first night home, I woke at 4am, turned my head to the right and immediately felt a sharp pain travelling down the left hand side of my neck and into my shoulder. I couldn't sleep after that, there was no position that was bearable.

'The pain didn't travel into my arm, but it became incredibly weak – too weak for me to drive or lift anything with it. My husband had been to a chiropractor before and he got in touch with him first thing in the morning.

'The chiropractor moved me around a lot to test how much movement I had, and how strongly I could resist his applying pressure on my joints. He tested my right and left side. Then I was given a heat treatment to losen the muscles. Next I lay down on my front and some embrocation was rubbed into the shoulder. He examined my pelvis and told me it was out of alignment and that one leg was 6.25 mm (¼ in) shorter than the other.

'His diagnosis was that I had a trapped nerve brought on by stress and abuse of my back with all the lifting I had done over the previous two weeks. He 'cracked' my pelvis and I nearly hit the roof! It wasn't painful at all but the cracking noise was quite terrifying. He worked his way up cracking my spine, my shoulder and my neck.

'Before treatment I couldn't turn my head around. Immediately after, I could turn it right round and look over my left shoulder. My neck felt a bit tender but I felt fantastic.'

CASE HISTORY
John, a mechanic, suffered from low- and mid-back pain for 18 months before he decided to try osteopathy to relieve the pain.

'I'm a lorry mechanic. It is a heavy physical job that obviously puts strain on your back. But for the last 20 years I've been into stock car racing which doesn't help either – it's like dodgems for grown-ups. The idea is to bash into the other cars. I've suffered from recurrent whiplash for years and although I've never broken any bones, I've got used to regular back pain. But eventually the pain got too bad to carry on. The osteopath explained what I was doing to my spine – she said it had aged more than it should have done for a man of my age. That was it. I gave up stock car racing (although I was gutted by the decision), and I now take more care at work.

'The treatment did hurt a bit, although she was trying to be as gentle as possible. But after four treatments I noticed a big difference. A lot of the pain had gone. After nine treatments I was 80% better, I'd definitely recommend it.'

HERBAL MEDICINE

There are two main strands of herbal medicine – Western and Chinese. Both work from the basic principle that the symptoms of illness are a sign of underlying disharmony and are the physical manifestations of the body's attempts to heal itself. The herbs prescribed by the practitioner help this self-healing process.

Our earliest ancestors recognized that plants could heal the body as well as nourish it and for most of history herbal medicine has been the most widely practised form of medication globally. The first Western herbal, written by Theophrastus dates back to 300 BC. The Chinese tradition is even more ancient.

A World Health Organization report in 1985 acknowledged that 80 per cent of the world's population live in developing countries and primarily depend on herbal medicine. Yet, in the West, since around the beginning of the eighteenth century, herbal medicine has been viewed by the medical profession as the uncouth poor relation – old-fashioned, unscientific, untested.

This hasn't prevented pharmaceutical companies from plundering the plant world for the active ingredients of our modern drugs. In 1985, it was estimated that 25 per cent of the active ingredients in modern drugs were plant-derived (1).

Slowly attitudes are changing and more doctors are being persuaded to refer their patients for herbal medicine, particularly when conventional treatments have failed.

How does it work?

Herbalism harnesses the 'life energy' of the plant to heal the depleted 'life energy' in our bodies, and the whole plant is used. This is in contrast to conventional medical drugs where the active ingredient of the plant is extracted. Herbal medicine uses the whole plant because of the concept of 'synergy' which reasons that the action of the whole plant is 'greater than the parts' and more beneficial to the body. A good example is the use of meadowsweet, which is prescribed for pain. The active ingredient of the plant is an aspirin-like chemical, but the whole plant also contains ingredients which 'buffer' the active ingredient, reducing the risk of the stomach irritation which is a side effect of aspirin.

Herbs are used to support the body in its fight against disease. But herbs also work to restore your body to health, by detoxifying it and strengthening your immune system so that your body's 'vital energy' will be able to cope with illness in the future.

You may view your symptoms as a nuisance; the herbalist will view them as your body's attempts to heal itself. Your symptoms are considered to be the body's self-healing mechanisms in action and in general should not be suppressed, but positively encouraged. So for some conditions be prepared for symptoms to get worse immediately after starting treatment. For instance, if part of your illness is a bad cough, the herbalist may prescribe a treatment which will encourage the cough with the aim of freeing up phlegm and clearing your respiratory tract more quickly.

Which ailments can it help?

Both doctors and patients have become more interested in the benefits of herbalism: doctors, because there has been a lot of progress in evaluating herbs' effectiveness by the standards of Western medicine so that they are more likely to accept the findings; patients, because of herbs' gentleness; this is especially important to parents of young patients. Western herbal treatments can help many minor ailments and have been found particularly helpful for urinary problems such as cystitis and digestive problems such as irritable bowel syndrome. Chinese herbal treatments can help such problems as arthritis, migraine, eczema and other skin disorders, hay fever, PMS and symptoms of the menopause.

WELL-RESPECTED HERBAL TREATMENTS

- **Dandelion leaf** This has proved to be as effective at eliminating water (via urine) as frusemide, one of the most commonly prescribed diuretic drugs. It has the advantage over frusemide as it replaces potassium lost in the urine.
- *Echinacea* This herb helps treat bacterial, viral and fungal infections and protects against colds and flu.
- **Feverfew** Taken regularly this herb will protect against migraine.
- **Garlic** Over a hundred research papers show that garlic lowers cholesterol, blood pressure and also helps to fight bacterial and viral infection.
- **Ginger** This can prevent nausea and sickness, morning sickness and prevents travel sickness if taken beforehand.
- *Ginkgo biloba* In Germany and France, extracts are amongst the most commonly prescribed drugs. It is used to help memory difficulties, dizziness, tinnitus, headaches, anxiety and some hearing problems.
- *Hypericum perforatum* (**St John's wort**) – the 'herbal Prozac'. Recent research in Germany has shown it to be as useful as commonly prescribed antidepressants. It also has antiviral properties.
- **Chinese herbs** These have succeeded in treating eczema which had proven stubborn in the face of conventional medicine. In a study with children a mixture of Chinese liquorice root and other herbs helped the skin condition and had no side effects.

What can you expect?

A Chinese herbalist uses the same theories, based on Taoism, that an acupuncturist uses (see pages 83–92). The herbalist will also make the same examinations and ask similar questions, which will include taking a case history, examining your face and tongue and taking your pulses.

Of all the complementary therapies, visiting a Western herbalist will be most like visiting your doctor, except that you will spend much more time with the herbalist. A thorough case history will be taken. He or she will want to know about the onset of the problem which has brought you there, how it started and what makes it worse or better. You will also have to give details of previous illnesses, health concerns (for instance, breathing difficulties or menstrual cramps), your work routine, stress factors, diet, exercise habits and any emotional factors you think might be relevant.

Western herbalists also use diagnostic tools you will recognize from your doctor's surgery. Your blood pressure will probably be taken and your eyes, ears or heart may be examined if the herbalist thinks it necessary. The herbalist may palpate (feel) your abdomen to assess how well your liver, bowels and other internal organs are working.

You will then be prescribed Western or Chinese herbs which come in a variety of forms.

● **Decoctions or 'soups'** You will be given a bag of roots, twigs or plants and strict instructions on how these should be boiled and simmered to form a drink. (Sometimes you are given powdered herbs that are diluted in boiling water.) You usually have to drink half a mugful or so, two or three times a day. These often taste and smell quite foul at first, but gradually become less offensive.

● **Tinctures** Western herbalists prescribe tinctures of herbs which are pure extracts of herbs diluted in an alcohol/water solution. Several may be mixed in one bottle to form a multi-prescription.

● **Creams or ointments** These are applied externally to soothe itching or irritating skin conditions.

● **Infusions** (herbs that are infused in water for 10 to 15 minutes, before straining and drinking.

● **Tablets**

How long does treatment take?

Acute (long-term) conditions such as a sore throat should respond to treatment very quickly, and with almost immediate improvement.

Chronic (long-term) problems will take longer. Most people who choose to visit a herbalist for the first time have a chronic condition which has not responded to conventional Western treatment and they are turning to herbalism as 'a last resort'. If this is the case you should be prepared for several follow-up sessions.

Herbalists see the symptoms of a disease as the attempts of the body to right itself. Merely curing the symptoms is therefore not the primary aim; a good herbalist will want to treat the underlying disease and so to restore balance to your body as a whole. All of this can take time to achieve. There may be underlying health problems that she believes are implicated in your primary illness and those will have to be tackled first. Like acupuncturists, herbalists may feel that dietary and/or lifestyle changes would benefit you, but knowing that this is difficult for most of us to implement, they won't expect you to make changes overnight, and will work with you to strengthen your system before suggesting these. You will probably see the herbalist at twice weekly intervals, at first and then three and four weekly intervals as you get better.

For advice on how to find a qualified herbalist see pages 149–150.

THE PRACTITIONER
Michael McIntyre is a practising herbalist.

'I'm all in favour of Western medicine and complementary medicine working together. But there is a fundamental difference between the way that orthodox medicine and complementary medicine works. Drugs can treat deep-rooted health problems amazingly quickly, much faster than herbalism works, but they don't address the real underlying reason for the illness. Illness is a warning: your body is trying to tell you there's a problem. I compare treating a problem with drugs to driving up to a red traffic light and in order to carry on with your journey getting out of the car and demolishing the traffic light to get rid of it. It's not always the most sensible solution. What we're trying to do with herbalism is to help people's systems to recover which can take a while. But for the patients it can be liberating – they're taking responsibility for their own health.'

CASE HISTORY

Diane, a slimming consultant, has suffered from excruciating migraine attacks most of her life.

'I've had migraines ever since I was 13, I'm 39 now. I've tried every drug going, and I've even had brain scans to try and find out the cause. The only time I've never suffered from them was when I was pregnant, but I remember that the very day after my first son was born I was blinded by a headache. It feels like a burning band is being pulled tight around my head. It starts over my right eye and spreads across the whole head. I get migraines every second day, sometimes every day.

'I decided to try herbal medicine because I was taking so many pills to try and control the pain. When you're in that much pain, you couldn't care less, you feel so bad you keep thinking, "Just two more might clear it". Then I started thinking, "What are all these drugs doing to my liver?" At first, I was sceptical of herbal medicine but I was impressed by my herbalist. If you believe in the person treating you, it really does help. I feel that he's really interested in me getting well.

'The herbal liquid tasted appalling, but you do get used to it. I've been having treatment now for a month and I'm not cured by any means, but there is an improvement and I have quite a lot of faith that I will be helped. Another interesting thing is that I've always been a perfectionist but now I'm more aware that I can let things go that aren't really important – I've become much less agitated.'

CASE HISTORY
Judy, a yoga teacher, used Chinese herbs for a skin condition.

'I'm a sun lover. I love to lie out in the sun. And because of sun exposure I got a kind of skin irritation – especially on my arms. They got very red and itchy. The doctor couldn't seem to do much, all that he would offer was steroid creams which I wasn't keen on. I went to see this Chinese herbalist who told me to avoid fish, cheese and sweet foods. He gave me a bag of what looked like grasses which I had to boil and infuse. This concoction looked awful and tasted vile, but within two weeks my skin condition had cleared up. It's now virtually disappeared although I still sunbathe. So far, so good.'

NUTRITIONAL MEDICINE

'We are what we eat': these days few of us would argue with this statement and that a healthy body requires a healthy diet. Nutritional medicine goes further and takes the converse view that an unhealthy body is partly due to an inadequate diet. Therapists aim to restore health by altering the body's biochemistry through dietary changes. The changes are determined by pinpointing whether an individual is suffering from vitamin or mineral deficiencies and whether certain foods are acting on his body as a mild poison.

A nutritional therapist should not be confused with a nutritionist (dietician). The latter work out a diet which will support the treatment being prescribed by a doctor or hospital physician. A nutritional therapist will decide on their own diagnosis of what is ailing you and from there will decide on a treatment programme.

It is something of a watchword that the Western world is over-fed but undernourished. Many experts now believe that our diet, which is high in fat, sugar and salt, and low in wholefoods and fresh produce, is in fact the major factor in causing the diseases which will kill most of us: cancer and heart disease.

But many of us are plagued day to day by minor symptoms, so minor that we accept them as routine: recurrent colds, persistent thrush, constant fatigue and niggling skin ailments. Nutritional therapists say that we don't need to suffer from these symptoms of low-grade bad health. Their view is that by modifying the body's biochemistry with dietary changes these symptoms can be eliminated.

Of course, the idea that 'food is our medicine' is a very ancient one, but much of our understanding of the importance of the chemical constituents of food in protecting against illness is relatively recent and there is a great deal of resistance to some of its ideas amongst physicians. As recently as the early 1980s, the eminent scientist and doctor, Linus Pauling, was openly ridiculed in at least one British medical school for his ideas that vitamin C could be used in the treatment of cancer.

What is accepted by everyone is that we cannot manufacture every nutrient that we need to stay alive. Human beings have to ingest a certain level of eight amino acids (the building blocks of protein), at least 13 vitamins and at least 19 minerals regularly in order to maintain body function. But when it comes to determining exactly how much of these nutrients we require, that is where the controversy arises.

Guidelines have been drawn up by governments, on the advice of expert committees, as to what these requirements should be. These values can vary widely, by as much as twenty-fold, from country to country. (Confusingly, in 1991, Great Britain replaced RDAs [Recommended Daily Allowances] with the near-identical DRVs [Dietary Reference Values] but we will continue to talk of RDAs as that's what appears on vitamin labels and in most of the literature.)

RDAs are the amounts which if ingested, will maintain life and prevent the development of specific diseases related to severe nutritional deficiency (for instance, scurvy which occurs from vitamin C deficiency).

However, RDAs have been described as the nutritional equivalent of the minimum wage – enough to maintain life but not enough to guarantee the quality of life. Adhering to them may not necessarily be enough to prevent nutrient deficiencies which lead to low-grade (and sometimes even severe) symptoms that interfere with our general sense of health and wellbeing. This becomes even more important if you take on board one of the fundamental concepts of nutritional therapy (and indeed one that it's hard to argue against); that of 'biochemical individuality'. In other words, we are all unique individuals, with unique requirements.

Put simply, your genetic, physiological, psychological and environmental influences dictate that the couple of glasses of orange juice and the mid-morning snack of fruit that you consume each day may well supply you with enough vitamin C to stay healthy. But that amount would be nowhere near sufficient for your hard-living, chain-smoking friend with a history of cancer in his family who lives in a more polluted part of the country.

There is another point worth making: although we are told repeatedly that a 'healthy, balanced' diet provides enough nutrients to supply our RDA levels for the day, how many people stick to a 'healthy, balanced' diet?

Very few, according to the research that has been done.

● The National Food Survey (Ministry of Agriculture, Fisheries and Food 1993) surveyed food diaries from 8,043 British households. The conclusion was that the average Briton is deficient in seven essential vitamins and minerals compared to the EC RDAs – the bare minimum recommended for maintaining health. These were: B1, B2, C and D; and minerals, zinc, magnesium and iron. Fifty per cent of the population were getting too little vitamin B6 and 40 per cent too little calcium. The MAFF survey showed that only one in 10 of us gets enough zinc, an especially important mineral for men as it plays a vital role in maintaining the health of sperm.

● American studies are just as worrying. The US Department of Agriculture, in 1981, reported that a significant percentage of the population receives well under 70 per cent of the US RDA for vitamins A, C and B plus cadmium, magnesium and iron. According to Dietary Intake Source Data for 1983, most typical diets have less than 80 per cent of the recommended intake of calcium, magnesium, iron, zinc, copper and manganese. Another US Department of Agriculture Survey, in 1989 reported that 90 per cent of US citizens fell below the RDA for chromium.

These are the bare minimum levels necessary to maintain health and most of us are failing to reach them. The vast majority of the population are very far from being in the state which nutritional therapists call 'optimum health'. Dr Emanuel Cheraskin, in 1974, promoted the idea of 'optimal dietary intake' – ingestion of nutrients at levels that produce above average health. Resulting from a 15-year study, Dr Cheraskin and his colleagues have established Suggested Optimal Nutrient Intake (SONIs) – nutrient intakes associated with optimal health. It is this state of optimal health which nutritional therapists aim to achieve.

The following table shows the RDAs (Recommended Daily Allowances) compared with SONIs (Suggested Optimal Nutrient Intake).

RDAs versus SONIS

Nutrient	RDA	SONI (under 50)
Vitamin A	800 µg	1000 µg
Vitamin C	60 mg	400 mg
Vitamin E	60 mg	400 mg
Vitamin B1	1.4 mg	7.5 mg
Vitamin B2	1.6 mg	2.5 mg
Vitamin B6	2 mg	10 mg
Folic acid	400 µg	800 µg

Over the age of 50, the SONIs double for Vitamins A, C and E and go up to 1000 µg for folic acid. B vitamin levels stay more or less constant.

The above table is based on the work of Dr Emanuel Cheraskin and his colleagues at the University of Alabama and their research of 13,500 people over a 15-year period.

How does it work?

A nutritional therapist is looking for several things when you first make a visit.

- A deficiency of vital vitamins and minerals.
- Food allergy or sensitivity. Nutritional therapists believe that between 20 and 80 per cent of people have some kind of allergy to food. Some of the common 'allergens' are wheat (gluten), cow's milk, eggs, yeast. If you are allergic to these foods, they are toxic to your body, and although our bodies can cope with them, the coping procedures result in symptoms of ill-health. Eliminating them from your diet gives your body a break from the stress of dealing with low-grade poisoning.

To take further strain off the body, nutritional therapists will usually recommend a diet rich in whole foods, low in processed foods and based as much as possible on organic produce. The theory (again, one hard to argue with) is that our food is less 'nutritious' than it used to be. Intensive farming procedures have leached vitamins from the soil so that vegetables haven't as high a vitamin and mineral content, and fruits are regularly sprayed with pesticides and preservatives. Pollution and farming methods mean that meat and fish aren't 'pure'. We are exposed to more chemicals through pesticides, preservatives and hormones than previous generations. We can also afford to drink more alcohol, smoke more tobacco and live in a much more polluted environment. Coping with all of us puts a strain on our bodies' excretory organs – primarily, the liver, kidney, lungs and skin.

Which ailments can it help?

Since good nutrition is fundamental to health just about any condition can benefit from dietary changes. However, if you are suffering from digestive problems especially irritable bowel syndrome (IBS), rheumatism and arthritis, skin disorders, PMS, candidiasis and a history of recurrent infections, then nutritional therapy may prove to be particularly useful.

There are many other conditions nutritional therapy can help, including the following.

● **Asthma** Levels of vitamin B6 in the body may be reduced in asthmatics (1). Where vitamin deficiency is established, treatment has been shown to reduce dramatically the frequency and duration of attacks. Asthmatic children given daily doses of vitamin B6 needed less drug intervention and saw improvement in symptoms.

There is evidence that a low magnesium intake may also be linked to asthma (2).

● **Cancer** Studies have shown that people who have a diet rich in beta carotene (the vegetable form of vitamin A, found especially in yellow and orange vegetables) are less likely to develop cancer, especially lung cancer. Doses of 60 mg for six months was found to reduce the risk of developing cancer of the mouth and throat in tobacco chewers in India (3).

Treating young women with cervical dysplasia (early signs of cervical cancer where cervical cells show signs of disruption) with 10mg of folic acid daily was found to clear up signs of early cancer in 100 per cent of patients (4). Young women with signs of early cervical cancer, given 10mg daily of folic acid for three months, showed significantly less progression in the disease process. In seven women the disease completely disappeared; four women who were given a placebo showed progression to full-blown cancer.

● **PMS** There is evidence that women suffering from PMS symptoms have less magnesium in their red blood cells. Magnesium supplements have been shown to alleviate premenstrual mood changes (5). Another study suggests that breast pain, weight gain, nervous tension and headache can also be successfully treated with magnesium supplementation although this was in an uncontrolled trial (that means the 192 women who took part were all given magnesium, none were given placebo so the power of suggestion can't be ruled out) (6).

● **Circulatory disease** There is now indisputable evidence of a link between the role vitamin E plays in protecting the heart and the peripheral circulatory system (7). Taking supplements has been shown to increase the 'goodie' cholesterol which helps prevent disease, to minimize the actions of the 'bad' cholesterol that causes it and to minimize the size of a heart attack. Eating a diet rich in vitamin E and other anti-oxidants may also help to reduce the risk of heart disease (8).

What can you expect?

There are several kinds of diagnostic procedures used by nutritional therapists. Some use laboratory tests – checking the blood and occasionally urine; hair or sweat samples can yield information on nutrient and hormone levels. Others use an electrical instrument known as the Vegatest machine. You hold a metal rod while the therapist tests a point on your skin for a changing electrical reaction to a whole host of common foodstuffs and well-known allergens (such as yeasts and pollens). You feel nothing while this is going on.

All therapists will take a thorough case history. You may be asked to fill in a questionnaire. The therapist will need details of your symptoms, medical history as well as that of your family; your diet; alcohol and cigarette consumption, exercise habits and all possible symptoms including very minor ones as they can build up to a clinical picture indicating a deficiency or toxicity. You may also be asked questions relating to your emotions, and how you respond to say, stress, and your answers can give significant clues.

Finally, based on the information gleaned from the consultation, the therapist will prescribe a diet tailored to your needs. You will almost certainly be asked to avoid certain foods or to include certain others in your diet. You may be given vitamin or mineral supplements to correct any deficiencies. Herbs are also often prescribed. These can be useful in detoxifiying specific organs.

During treatment you will probably be asked to eat a diet rich in wholefoods, fruit, vegetables and to avoid processed foods, tea, coffee and soft drinks. Nutritional therapists are often fussy about water, recommending that you avoid tap water and drink bottled or filtered water. All of these measures mean that the body doesn't have to work so hard at processing and can 'focus' its energies on healing your body.

How long does treatment take?

This depends on how long you have been suffering from symptoms, how well you respond to treatment and not least, how careful you are in following the recommended programme. Nutritional therapy takes two to three months to really 'bite' and patients need to visit the therapist every two to three weeks.

Anyone considering nutritional therapy should be aware that practically no other therapy 'interferes' so much with your normal routine, as you often have to make quite profound changes to the way you eat, and therefore, live. Some strong people find that they can keep to the programme with little effort, but for others it's far more difficult. You will almost certainly have to eat in a rather strange way and it can make socializing, in particular, difficult. Therapists are conscious of problem and the good ones will try to make the transition as easy as possible for you by introducing the changes to your diet gradually.

For advice on how to find a qualified nutritional therapist see page 153.

THE PRACTITIONER
Dr Sarah Myhill, a doctor, uses nutritional medicine alongside orthodox medicine in her practice.

'I got frustrated because drugs weren't always curing a patient's problems – they were just managing the symptoms. I kept asking myself, "Why is this person ill" and it seemed to me that it must come down to body biochemistry. That's why I got interested in nutritional medicine. I started treating patients with irritable bowel syndrome (IBS), and then Crohn's disease. I've found migraine and chronic fatigue syndrome (CFS) respond well, too.

'It's well recognized in farm animals that if there is a fertility problem the answer is often a mega dose of vitamins, so I got involved with Foresight (see pages 60–61) and tried to help patients attempting to conceive. That's worked well, too.

'The patients have to put some effort in but the treatment is so effective and so safe that many of them are happy to do it.

And of course, nutritional medicine cures – so it is very cost-effective for the NHS.'

CASE HISTORY
Polly, a business woman, had her first baby at aged 43.

'When I got married three years ago, we knew we wanted to have a baby right away. Because of my age, it seemed sensible to do all we could to help. I had heard about Foresight and we saw one of their doctors. She tested us with a Vegatest machine to pinpoint nutritional deficiencies. Generally, we were healthy, although she did pick up some kind of electromagnetic energy coming from both of us, and suggested we change our bed. She asked me to avoid beef, dairy products, caffeine and alcohol and I decided myself to stop using pesticides in the garden. The whole plan is geared towards both partners living the healthiest life they can.

'It took two years for me to conceive and sometimes I felt incredibly negative and miserable. I also went for acupuncture at that time which I found immensely helpful. It boosted my morale, helped counterbalance a lot of emotional stress I was under, and I think it was crucial in fine-tuning my system to allow me to conceive.'

CASE HISTORY
Jack has a demanding job in advertising which began to affect his health.

'My work is very stressful. I'm always flying from place to place and I work at the weekends. Then suddenly I began to develop muscle twitches, my sleep suffered and I was incredibly lethargic. I thought I was developing ME.

'I went to see a doctor who knew about ME but also practised nutritional medicine. The doctor ran some tests and told me

I had a magnesium deficiency. I follow a good diet anyway but apparently magnesium deficiency is quite common and stress depletes our stores of it even more.

'Within a few days I had dramatically improved and in four months my symptoms had completely gone.

'I like to work hard and it was appalling when I was operating below par. But I have cut down on the travelling and have found that although I still work hard I respond much better to stress now.'

HEALING

Healing fascinates us. Religions have been founded on it, and the course of many people's lives has been changed by it. Little wonder that it has been subjected to more scientific investigation than all the other complementary medicines put together (except perhaps for hypnosis). There are cave drawings of healing sessions in existence and the first written record of healing appeared over 5,000 years ago. Every culture in the world has used it. But we still cannot explain how it works, although there is plenty of evidence that healers have the power to initiate definite changes at a molecular level, whether or not you believe that the power they have is divinely given.

Put simply, an interaction appears to take place between the energy fields of the healer and the person being healed. The person's energy is rebalanced through the focused attention of the healer. Nearly always the person experiences a feeling of deep relaxation. The healer treats physical symptoms, such as pain, and also unblocks any emotional stress in the body which may be contributing to the illness. The body is 'freed' up so that self-healing is activated.

Of course, patients who have exhausted all other forms of therapy may seek spiritual healing hoping for a 'miracle'. Although miracles have taken place, they are not common. But even when there is no cure, terminal patients often receive much relief from healing.

Central to the idea of healing is 'focused intention'. By passing hands over the patient or sometimes by 'laying on of hands', the healer acts as a conduit whereby the healing can be channelled to the patient. The concentration necessary to effect healing can be intense.

There is evidence that the energy healers draw on is open to us all. For one study, 32 nurses were trained in the methods employed by a healer and they acted as healers in the research. However, although the energy may be there for anyone to tap into, to become a healer seems to take certain clear personality traits. Psychological testing of the nurses selected to take part confirmed that they were of the 'self-actualized' personality type: people with a strong sense of themselves and their purpose in life. Ghandi, Nelson Mandela and the Dalai Lama are good examples of self-actualized people.

Even if you have not had healing, you may have been the recipient of what is known as the 'therapeutic touch'; often the best doctors, nurses and complementary therapists use touch every working day to reassure and comfort patients, and many of them actively train to expand their ability to heal through touch (see page 19).

However, there is no doubt that some people have extraordinary, innate healing ability. Healers say that it is not they who heal, but that they are merely channels for a greater energy. Some believe their gift is God-given; others prefer not to explain their ability through religion. Certainly, the person being healed does not have to have any religious faith to receive benefit. He does not even have to believe in the healer, much less in a God. All that is necessary is that the person wants to be healed and is open to letting the healing take place.

There are upwards of 7,000 registered healers in Great Britain. Many of them work with doctors, a surprising number of whom are happy to refer patients to healers having themselves seen proof of healing in action which they could not explain with medical science.

How does it work?

We don't know, but studies have shown healers can affect the physical properties of inanimate objects suggesting that they are emanating energy of some sort. Extrapolating from these findings gives us some ideas of how healers' energy works to heal the body.

In one study, a well-known (now deceased) healer, Olga Worrall, treated containers of copper salt solutions as if she were undertaking a healing. The crystals obtained from these solutions were coarser than the crystals obtained from water treated exactly the same way minus the healing. Further measurement showed changes consistent with an alteration in the hydrogen bonds of the 'healed' water (1).

Another study showed that 'healed' water became polarized, and polarized water has been shown to stimulate plant growth (2).

The conclusions of the study with the 32 nurses (mentioned on page 121) was that healing can increase haemoglobin levels thereby transporting more oxygen to the cells (3).

Finally, healing has been shown to heal humans more quickly than would be expected, even when the healer never meets the patients. In a famous study, subjects agreed to having a cut made on their skin – all the cuts were of the same depth and length. Half the group received healing at a distance (the healer focused on their healing) and half did not. Those being healed were not told that they were part of an experiment into healing so that they could not be accused of being open to suggestion. After 8 and 16 days the wounds were examined and on both dates, the wounds of the group receiving healing were smaller than the group who had not experienced any healing treatment at all (4).

Who can it help?

Research has shown that it is helpful for pain, anxiety, wound healing, for speeding up the rehabilitation process after any injury, headaches, high blood pressure, stress-related illnesses and symptoms of these including insomnia.

Because the effects can sometimes be very powerful, extra care should be taken with the very young, the old and frail, patients who have experienced shock and pregnant women. This does not mean they cannot have healing, but shorter periods may be advisable especially on the first consultation.

What can you expect?

The room where you are treated will almost certainly have a relaxed atmosphere and there may be soothing music playing. The healer will probably spend some time talking to you about your illness and finding out about you before the healing proper begins. You may remain seated during the healing, or be asked to lie on a couch.

Clothing is not removed although you will probably be asked to take off your shoes.

The healer will take a few minutes to 'attune' to you and focus on your problems. Some healers lay their hands on you; others pass their hands over you, just above your body.

Patients report different experiences. You may feel nothing. You may experience heat, tingling or coldness where the healer's hands pass. The most common feeling reported is one of intense relaxation and loss of all sense of time – a healing session that lasts an hour, seems to go by in a few minutes. Usually the healing lasts between 15 minutes and an hour. The average time for a whole session is usually about an hour.

How long does treatment take?

For most simple aches and pains, usually only a couple of sessions are needed. With other more serious conditions, healers would expect improvement after six sessions but it needs to be given time.

For advice on how to find a qualified healer see page 149.

THE PRACTITIONER
Geoff is a healer.

'I believe that we all have the ability to heal ourselves. We've cut off the mind from the body but the mind is very powerful and what we've lost is a powerful contact. The ability I've got potentially exists in other people. They just don't know it. I teach them how to access it.

'I help people who are physically sick, but also those who need spiritual upliftment. By affecting their electomagnetic energy, I change the way they see themselves. Even in cases where their illness isn't totally curable they learn how to deal with it differently.'

CASE HISTORY
Linda, a housewife, was in a bad car accident which she doesn't believe she completely had come to terms with until she had healing.

'The accident meant I had to have my spleen removed and my pelvis and wrists were fractured. I nearly died. Because of the accident I had an out of body experience, but I never told anyone. I think my family and friends would have had me locked up if I had started talking about it!

'I suppose that experience has made me quite open to new ideas, but it was years and years after the accident before I found myself going to a healer and I found it an extraordinary experience. I felt energy coming down my spine and I felt lighter and much happier. People I have known all my life can see a change in me and I can also see from their attitude towards me that I've changed. I'm a happier person and a better mother. I'm now much calmer and less judgemental.'

CLINICAL ECOLOGY
(Environmental Medicine)

None of us lives in a bubble. Each day we come across any number of what clinical ecologists would call 'environmental challenges' and how we cope with these challenges, to a large extent, determines how healthy we remain.

Clinical ecology (or to give it its more exact description, environmental medicine) is the branch of medicine which identifies these stressors and, once recognized, helps the patient deal with them.

It is the medicine of allergy. It is also a fairly new medicine (although it had its beginnings in the last century) because it is based on a thorough understanding of body biochemistry which is in itself, a fairly new science. As our knowledge of biochemistry grows, we understand more. It is often practised in this country by doctors who have specialized in the treatment of allergies, but other therapists, notably those in nutritional medicine also use many of the same techniques. However, despite its acceptance by some doctors, many of its ideas are still on the 'fringe' of conventional medicine although in other European countries they have a wider acceptance (and no doubt, we will have it here too, in the future).

Clinical ecologists see health as dependent on our individual ability to withstand a whole host of low-grade environmental challenges. Our genes, how well we are to begin with, our nutritional state, our psychological make-up – all of these combine to form our 'adaptive capacity' and this in turn determines how well we will fight off environmental challenges that we meet.

The lower our adaptive capacity, the more likely we are to fall ill. Environmental challenges include foods, temperature and humidity, electromagnetic fields, radiation, toxins (in the air, food, water and environment), drugs, noise, stress of all kinds and bacterial and viral infection.

How does it work?

The clinical ecologist will need to do tests to try and identify allergic triggers. He can then give advice to patients on how to handle or prevent the symptoms.

In the case of food allergy/intolerance, this is a complicated procedure. It usually involves elimination diets. These are usually one of two types.

● You follow a very limited diet consisting of foods unlikely to cause allergies, such as rice, lamb, vegetables and pears, and gradually reintroduce foods to see if they provoke a reaction. This is a big undertaking and would only be suggested either when there are multiple foods causing problems or when symptoms are severe.
● You eat a normal diet but eliminate the foods suspected of causing the allergy. They are introduced later to confirm whether or not you are allergic to them.

When the allergy is due to house dust mites, advice is centred on eliminating them as much as possible from the home. They lurk in soft furnishings and changing the bedding, flooring and furniture can help. There are also special cleaning fluids which can kill them. An allergy that is caused by moulds and fungi often goes unrecognized. This is usually made worse by damp environments such as cellars and greenhouses, or when undertaking a task like sweeping up leaves. Again, clinical ecologists can determine the extent of any allergy and advise accordingly.

Often an allergic reaction has multiple triggers. When this is the case and/or simple avoidance isn't possible, (say, in the case of pollen during the hay fever season) a clinical ecologist can try desensitization. This means introducing small amounts of the allergen to the body over a period of time. If successful, this can decrease or even banish symptoms.

Treating the allergy itself may not be enough if it is due to an underlying disease. The clinical ecologist can also identify if such a condition exists. For example the following may be present:

● Dysbiosis, where there is a change in the normal bacterial growth in the gut, is often associated with an overgrowth of the fungus *Candida albicans*. This can lead to a phenomenon known as 'leaky gut' when toxins break through the gut wall and cause widespread symptoms and a general feeling of being unwell. The clinical ecologist can treat the imbalance in bacteria and any existing candidiasis (see pages 42–45).

● A whole host of nutritional deficiencies can contribute to allergies. For instance, vitamin B6 has been shown to help sensitivity to monosodium glutamate (MSG) found in food, notably Chinese. Sensitivity to sulphite, again often used in food preparation, can be blocked by taking vitamin B12.

● Multiple sensitivities can develop after a severe viral infection because of disturbance to the immune system. The patient may be suffering from chronic fatigue syndrome.

● A whole new area of medicine is opening up called psychoneuroimmunology which recognizes the important part that our psychological make-up plays on our immune system. Increasingly, it seems that many sensitivities may be linked to our state of mind.

Which ailments can it help?

Many chronic (long-term) illnesses can be cured by visiting a clinical ecologist. The following are the main ones.

- **Asthma** This is often triggered by food allergies and intolerances as well as house dust mites, pets, pollens and moulds, chemicals and exhaust fumes.
- **Migraine** About 75 per cent of patients have been helped by elimination diets. Besides foods, chemicals (including chlorine), exhaust fumes and tobacco smoke can also cause migraine.
- **Rheumatoid arthritis** Seventy-three per cent of patients in one study reported feeling better following an elimination diet (1).
- **Eczema** This can be caused by cows' milk, wheat, citrus fruits and tomatoes and house dust mites.
- **Hyperactivity** Colourings, preservatives, cows' milk, cheese, chocolate, wheat, oranges and sugar have all been linked to hyperactivity problems.
- **Bowel disease** Studies show that up to 70 per cent of patients with irritable bowel syndrome can be helped by changing their diet (2). Cutting out certain foods can also help Crohn's disease.

What can you expect?

When you visit a clinical ecologist she will take a careful case history. Special emphasis is placed on when you first experienced the symptoms and how extreme they were, so that she can build up a chronological picture of your allergic history. She will want to know about the foods you eat (especially those eaten frequently or regularly), smoking habits, drugs including any past intolerances), any allergy to pets, susceptibility to infections or details of a family history of allergies.

Clinical ecologists use a whole battery of tests to help them diagnose sensitivity. Most involve testing small amounts of suspected allergens on the skin or tongue, by injection or by inhalation, and noting any allergic reactions that result.

The Vegatest machine, widely used in Germany and becoming more common here may be used. You hold a metal rod while the therapist tests a point on your skin (an acupuncture trigger point, usually on your foot or finger) for a changing electrical reading when a whole host of common foodstuffs and well-known allergens (such as yeasts) are introduced into the system. It is completely painless, and is about 70 to 80 per cent accurate at detecting intolerances or allergies.

When intolerance to a certain food (or foods) is suspected, the clinical ecologist will discuss dietary options with you.

How long does treatment take?

It's impossible to say. It can take some time to identify the allergies positively, and in the case of food sensitivities, restricted diets will have to be followed for some weeks before confirmation can be made that the allergy or intolerance exists. If desensitization is considered worthwhile, treatment can take even longer. However, if the therapist is on the right lines, you should feel better fairly rapidly after following the treatment programme. Within weeks, even days, you should start to see an improvement in your symptoms.

It is an essential part of treatment that you feel confident in the therapist. There are sadly many cases of patients who have struggled through months of following restricted diets with absolutely no benefit. Sadly, by the time they realize that there is unlikely ever to be any benefit, they have parted with a good deal of money.

Prescribing the best treatment can be a difficult process and there is never a guarantee of a cure, but clinical ecology is based largely on scientific investigation and knowledge. It is not enough for the therapist to have a vague feeling that you are suffering from a certain disease, or a certain allergy which is based on a description of your symptoms and little else. Testing and elimination have to be essential parts of the process.

For advice on how to find a qualified clinical ecologist see pages 148–149.

THE PRACTITIONER
Dr Julian Kenyon is a practising clinical ecologist.

'I use nutritional and environmental medicine as well as acupuncture, homoeopathy, herbalism and psychology. I believe that when patients come to you at the end of the road with nothing else to turn to, the most important quality you can offer them is creativity and imagination in helping them solve their particular problem. Evidence-based medicine is so rigid. Patients should feel that their practitioner can think creatively about their problem in a relevant way.'

CASE HISTORY
Roy, unemployed, has had Chronic Fatigue Syndrome for the last five years.

'Five years ago I went on holiday to Tunisia. On the second week I got really bad food poisoning. It might have been salmonella but the doctors can't be sure. The result was that I got internal bleeding and suspected ulcerative colitis. I was given steroids and antibiotics and everything healed up, but it was then thought I hadn't had ulcerative colitis at all. I felt awful, drained of energy and depressed. Even getting out of bed and taking a shower completely exhausted me.

'I used to have my own business, but it was impossible for me to work and for the last five years I've had to concentrate on getting well. I've tried all sorts of things: elimination diets, jin shin jyutsu (which is a form of energy balancing), reflexology and aromatherapy, spiritual healing and regression therapy. They all helped a bit. I'd get overexcited thinking that I'd found a cure but then I'd relapse. I'm now seeing a doctor who is a clinical ecologist. He diagnosed me as being low in minerals, especially magnesium. He is giving me injections which aren't very pleasant. I'm also taking supplements as I'm low on vitamins A and B and zinc. I like the fact that he is confident he can help me but doesn't give me any guarantees. The first thing I noticed was that I was sleeping better – better than I've done in years and I'm not so tired, but it will be a long haul until I'm completely well. However, I'm optimistic about the future.'

MIND–BODY THERAPIES
(Yoga, Meditation, Hypnotherapy, Qigong)

Western medicine is the only branch of medicine that does not have at the heart of its teaching the idea that the mind is linked inextricably to the body and that the one profoundly affects the other. We do accept that illness of the body can negatively affect our mental state, but it is only very recently that we have accepted the possibility of the converse; that our mind, spirit and mental attitude could result in disease of the body. On the other hand, the traditional Chinese approach is that mind, body and emotions are one integrated whole. Emotions cause physical illness, and disease of the organs results in emotional vulnerability.

A practitioner of Traditional Chinese Medicine, faced with a female patient complaining of a stiff hip, is likely to think that the most important part of the treatment plan is to help the patient overcome her understandable fear and distress as a result of a burglary she endured six months earlier. Due to restrictions on his time, a Western doctor would write a prescription for anti-inflammatories to alleviate the symptoms without ever discovering their cause – that his patient had been burgled.

Now it is readily accepted that chronic stress and an unbalanced lifestyle can affect the function of specific organs. It makes perfect sense that steps taken to relax, to develop a positive outlook and to achieve a sense of inner calm can result in a positive improvement in health. Since 1955, when the British Medical Association accepted hypnotherapy as a valid treatment, mind–body therapies have increasingly been perceived by Western doctors as useful in treating certain diseases.

The Sanskrit word for yoga ('yuj') means 'to bind' and that is what mind–body therapies aim to do; to bind mind, body and spirit into a harmonious whole. In the West, we treat illness as the 'enemy'; the mind–body approach is to see illness as a message that we have overlooked something on a physical, emotional or spiritual level and that it needs our attention. The aim of treatment is to heal and strengthen the whole. The mind can have an extraordinarily powerful effect on the body, and mind–body therapies harness that special power to heal.

Mind–body therapies work primarily by releasing tension and inducing feelings of relaxation.

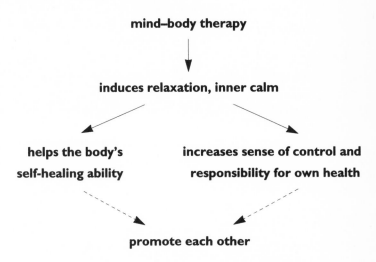

Which ailments can they help?

As more research is carried out, it is clear that all of us would benefit from learning to relax properly. Meditation, yoga and qigong are practised by millions on a daily basis to achieve clarity of thought, the ability to relax at will, and to prevent disease in the future. Arguably it is as a preventative form of medicine that they offer us the most.

These are the therapeutic applications, backed up by clinical evidence:

● **Chronic pain** Hypnotherapy has been shown to help relieve headaches, nerve pain, sciatica, arthritis and menstrual pain in one study of 178 patients. Six months later 78 per cent were still pain free; 44 per cent after two years and 36.5 per cent after three years (1). Pain is perceived by the mind and the mind can be trained to perceive pain as having diminished. It can help with all conditions where pain is a nuisance.

● **Long-term pain** An eight-week programme of meditation helped 61 per cent of patients with long-term pain achieve at least a 50 per cent reduction; a further 22 per cent of patients achieved at least a 33 per cent reduction (2).

● **Irritable bowel syndrome** Hypnotherapy has had dramatic results in chronic (long-term) IBS which hasn't responded to anything else. In one study, all patients aged 50 or under were cured (see page 36).

● **Anxiety** Hypnotherapy and meditation are well proven to help with anxiety. Cancer patients taught meditation report feeling less anxious and depressed as well as suffering less pain and discomfort.

● **Phobias and addiction** These conditions have been found to respond very well to hypnotherapy.

● **High blood pressure** Meditation has been proven to lower high blood pressure. The meditative technique doesn't have to be elaborate to work (see the boxes on pages 136 and 137) (3).

● **Asthma** Patients suffering from asthma respond well to hypnotherapy, needing less medication and fewer hospital admissions (4). Patients who did yoga for 65 minutes daily needed less drugs and hospital intervention than a group who controlled their asthma only with drugs (5).

Hypnotherapy

Hypnotherapy induces a deeply relaxed state in which the patient (although never helpless to resist) is highly susceptible to suggestions from the therapist. What suggestions are given depends on the aim of treatment, for example, that the patient feel less pain, be more relaxed, stop smoking, or think more positively about their illness.

Possibly no therapy has attracted so much malevolent press as hypnotherapy. Only recently, papers have been full of reports of people hypnotized during stage shows claiming to be still suffering emotional trauma years afterwards. Hypnosis is 'magical' and this reputation has arguably done it more harm than good. It is a highly effective therapy, but can also be highly entertaining. The original hypnotherapist, Mesmer, dazzled late seventeenth-century audiences with his ability to heal. But unfortunately his love of putting on a good show led to his earning the contempt of physicians of the day and ever since hypnotherapists have had to put up with claims of being charlatans at best and dangerous at worst.

Clearly and emphatically it should be stated that in the hands of a trained hypnotherapist you are perfectly safe. You will be encouraged to enter a trance-like state, but even in that state you are always fully aware of what is going on and you cannot be made to do anything that you are uncomfortable with. You can 'wake-up' at any time. There is no such thing as staying 'under' after the session. You may feel relaxed but you will certainly not remain under the hypnotherapist's influence, or be still in the trance-like state after the session is ended.

HOW DOES IT WORK?

Hypnotherapy works by calming the conscious mind so that it 'closes down' and your whole concentration is focused on the ideas which the hypnotherapist is suggesting to you. There are several levels of this trance-like state. In the deepest level, the patient feels no pain (it is this level that is used for operations conducted without an anaesthetic). However, only between 20 to 30 per cent of the population are able to go this 'deep'. It is in the lesser trance-like states that most hypnotherapy takes place. At this level, your body functions may slow down, you will be deeply relaxed and your eyes will be closed. You are so open to the hypnotherapist's suggestions that you are able to carry out actions which would normally be impossible. For instance, the hypnotherapist may suggest to you that you hold your arm above your head and you would be able to do so, comfortably, for a long period of time, far longer than you could in your normal state.

The World Health Organization has estimated that 90 per cent of us can reach this state and therefore can be hypnotized successfully. How effective the hypnotherapy is, however, depends on how open the patient is to hypnotic suggestions when their conscious mind 'switches on' again. The suggestions usually have to be reinforced by the therapist at further sessions and by the patient themselves in-between sessions.

WHAT CAN YOU EXPECT?

Your therapist should be someone you feel comfortable with. It's especially important in hypnotherapy that you have a rapport with the therapist. The consulting room will probably be calm and relaxed, and quiet. Distracting noise doesn't help. Part (or all of the first session) is taken up with the therapist getting to the root of your problem. You will then be asked to lie on a couch or remain seated in a comfortable chair. In a hypnotic state you will appear to be sleeping deeply, when in fact, you are awake. To help you enter the trance, the therapist may ask you to imagine a peaceful scene in detail, and then ask you what you can feel, hear and touch. Often you are asked to descend a staircase in your imagination, counting down the steps. While in the trance, the hypnotist will make suggestions to benefit your healing (all of these will be discussed in full with you prior to the session).

Then you will be guided out of the trance, perhaps by walking up the steps counting yourself 'up'. The final words are usually along the lines of 'When I count to three you will wake up, you will remember everything that has been said to you. You will feel relaxed and refreshed.' The session usually lasts between one hour and an hour and a half. Some therapists will be happy to let you tape the session so you can play it back to yourself between appointments.

HOW LONG DOES TREATMENT TAKE?

For a simple problem such as trying to give up smoking, usually four to six weekly sessions will be needed. Benefit should be expected after this amount of sessions whatever the problem although as many as 12 sessions may be needed.

For advice on how to find a qualified hypnotherapist see page 152.

THE PRACTITIONER
Dr Peter Whorwell, a gastroenterologist has pioneered the treatment of IBS with hypnotherapy.

'I'm a very pragmatic physician. I like a nice direct approach. The mind affects the muscles under voluntary control, so I wondered if it could affect the muscles which aren't under our control like those in the gut. And it can. When we selected the patients we thought most suitable, we had a 100 per cent success rate, but now we take referrals from all over the country and some of patients aren't always going to get along as well with hypnosis so our success rate has dropped to about 75 per cent. The patient has to be willing to try and to practise. We can't make someone better – they make themselves better. All hypnosis is self-healing.'

CASE HISTORY
Eric is a catering manager who started having stomach problems four years ago.

'You can't afford to be ill in my line of work, but it's very stressful. When I started feeling pain in my stomach and passing blood I went along to the doctor because I thought that it might be cancer. I have high blood pressure and he thought it might be the tablets that I was taking which were causing the pain. The doctor also gave me some leaflets on irritable bowel syndrome (IBS). I discovered that I had all the symptoms of IBS, so eventually we concluded that was what it was.

'He said that IBS can be cured by hypnotherapy and that he would refer me if I was interested. I would have done anything to get rid of the pain, the bloated feeling and wind which was really uncomfortable.

'The sessions at the beginning were all about relaxing, and I was given a tape which I have to play every day. Now after four sessions he's got onto me visualizing controlling my gut. I had to describe to the hypnotist what my pain feels like. It's like a tennis ball so now I've got to imagine shooting it like a clay pigeon.

'It has helped me a lot already. I'm hyperactive but I've become a lot calmer. I used to wake up about two or three times in the night. Now I play the tape before bed if I can and I don't wake at all during the night. I've never been more relaxed. It's brilliant. You have to give 200 per cent and do exactly what they tell you. I've got another eight sessions to go, but so far so good.'

MEDITATION

During meditation you simply calm the mind so that it becomes pleasantly focused on the present moment, neither reacting to memories from the past, nor being preoccupied with plans for the future. For best results it should be carried out as often as possible, and ideally on a daily basis, for about 5–10 minutes initially, building up to 20.

You can meditate in one of two ways.

● Concentrating – on a word, your breath, a mark on the wall or a candle flame. Whenever thoughts intrude, you should bring your attention back to the object of concentration.
● Mindfulness – allowing thoughts to drift through the mind, not reacting to them, but acknowledging them before letting them drift off again.

Meditating has been shown to decrease the heart rate, blood pressure, regulate the breathing rate, affect the hormone levels and relax tense muscles. There is also a change in the pattern of brain waves while meditating.

Those who practise meditation regularly report increased concentration, clarity of thought and peace of mind.

THE RELAXATION RESPONSE

Dr Herbert Benson, Professor of Medicine at Harvard Medical School is convinced that quiet inactivity is just as important to long-term good health as exercise. Studies of his patients has shown that their ability to recover depended again and again on: 'the exercising of their beliefs, values, thoughts and feelings . . . their spirit as much as their muscles'. He developed what he called the 'relaxation response', a very simple form of meditation. As well as calming your mind, when you practise you will lower your blood pressure and heart rate, breathing and metabolic rate.

● Pick a focus word or short phrase which has peaceful connotations such as 'love', 'calm' or 'relax'.

● Sit somewhere which is comfortable and quiet, preferably use the same place each time.

● Close your eyes and consciously relax all your muscles.

● Breathe slowly and naturally, and each time you breathe out repeat your focus word silently.

● Be passive. Don't worry about how well you are doing. When other thoughts come to mind, just dismiss them and return to the word repetition.

● Continue doing this for 10–20 minutes.

● Don't stand up immediately. Let other thoughts return to your mind, and then sit still for another minute before rising.

Practise this simple meditation once every day or ideally twice daily, morning and night.

QIGONG

Qigong means 'energy cultivation' and along with acupuncture and herbalism forms one of the bases of Traditional Chinese Medicine. Around 60 million people are thought to practise Qigong on a regular basis as a means of calming their minds and improving their health.

Qigong has been described as 'meditation in motion' and has similar benefits to the health as meditation. Slow graceful movements regulate the body, while controlled breathing and visualization methods help to regulate the mind. The aim is to improve the circulation of the human bioelectrical field and as the name implies, stimulate the flow of energy in the body – Qi (or Chi).

Chinese studies report that qigong has helped asthma, arthritis, gastrointestinal disorders, insomnia, pain, depression, anxiety, cancer, coronary heart disease and AIDS. It has also been claimed that certain mental conditions are rarer in China because so many of the population practise Qigong. These claims have not been substantiated by Western studies, but Qigong is a superb preventative health measure promoting suppleness and peace of mind. It is a great substitute for people who find it hard to meditate but want to experience the benefits.

Yoga

This exercise movement is a method of promoting healing by encouraging the flow of energy through the body via certain specific movements known as postures. Some of these don't look easy to achieve, but generally they are not difficult. It's not necessary to achieve a full lotus or headstand to get benefit. It is recommended to take yoga classes, however, as it is important to learn the postures properly. These postures are designed to make the body supple and allow the better flow of the 'life force' around the body. Yoga has specific therapeutic benefits, and it is also an excellent preventative health measure.

HOW DOES IT WORK?

Yoga also helps calm the mind and acts as a form of meditation. Mentally it relaxes the mind, helps control stress, and seems to banish negative thoughts. Central to this is yoga breathing. Mostly we breathe too shallowly from the upper chest. Yoga requires deep breathing from the diaphragm which increases energy and improves body circulation.

Classes are relaxed affairs. Wear loose clothing. The teacher will take you through some warm-up postures and breathing exercises before moving on to proper postures. Don't strain yourself, but just take yoga at your own pace. The aim is to perform the postures slowly and smoothly. Unlike normal exercise classes, the postures all flow into one another. At the end there is always a relaxation period so that you leave the class feeling relaxed and refreshed.

HOW LONG DOES YOGA TAKE?

You will probably feel better after one session but regular practice is needed to get full benefit. Yoga is most useful if practised every day, although after you have learned the postures you can do them at home between classes. Yoga is said to be most therapeutic if practised in the early morning.

For advice on finding the right yoga teacher see pages 152–153.

THE PRACTITIONER
Kitty Kennedy is a practising yoga therapist.

'Everything is about energy. I feel illness and disease are the physical representation of energy flow being disturbed or blocked. Put simply, yoga can help remove these blocks, improve circulation, body functioning and breathing. Yoga balances the mind, body and spirit but that may sound too "new age" for some people so I tend to concentrate on the physical. We can't all spend our lives sitting under trees and meditating, but we can all seek balance for our bodies.'

CASE HISTORY
Jean, an administrator, used yoga to help recover her health.

'I had a pretty stressful job as an administrator and I don't suppose I was particularly happy in my job at that time. I got bronchial pneumonia when I got back from my honeymoon. We had been touring around in a car and the doctor said one more day on the road and I would have had to go to hospital. This illness was a devastating experience. I was terribly weak and breathless and felt like an elderly person. Walking up one staircase knocked me out. I was just 35 at the time. I went to see a homoeopath who helped me begin to recover and he suggested I take yoga classes to help my breathing.

'I started going to yoga classes once a week. After six months I felt pretty well. The body work helped my physical symptoms but it also calmed my mind. My teacher decided not to teach classes any more so I continued seeing her on a private basis. I practise Hatha yoga and it works just like a prescription of medicine. I haven't had any recurrence of the bronchial symptoms and it's helped improve my whole life and outlook beyond recognition.'

4 finding a therapist

FINDING A THERAPIST THROUGH YOUR DOCTOR

You may be surprised to discover that on the whole doctors are very open to complementary medicine. Some brand new research, as yet unpublished, claims that as many as 93 per cent of doctors in Great Britain have referred patients to a therapist and that 40 per cent of them offer some form of treatment through the National Health Service. Around 6 per cent of patients receiving complementary therapy have it funded by the NHS.

The treatments covered in this book are the ones most likely to receive NHS funding with the exception of nutritional medicine. However, as has been pointed out, there is a grey area between clinical ecology and nutritional medicine. Clinical ecologists can counsel in nutritional medicine and many are medically trained (indeed we recommend you try to find one that is). Some work privately, but they may take NHS patients in which case your doctor could refer you.

There are also doctors who have a special interest in nutritional medicine and prescribe supplementation rather than drugs. They are likely to be a member of the British Society for Nutritional Medicine in which case the Society may be able to tell you if such a doctor is working in your area, and get a referral from your doctor.

In the case of homoeopathy there are five NHS-funded homoeopathic hospitals in Great Britain (see pages 150–151) to which you can be referred by your doctor.

Of course, your doctor may have different therapists working within your own practice, in which case, if he thinks you a suitable case for treatment, he can refer you to them. This is far more likely if your doctor is a fund-holder (see box on page 143). Theoretically, any doctor, fundholding or not, can refer his or her patients to a complementary therapist, but lately, cutbacks mean that it is more unlikely. With non-fundholding doctors, the referrals are usually to a local centre or unit which is using complementary therapy, for instance to an acupuncturist connected to a rheumatology unit, but unfortunately many of these have now closed.

Dr Ian Smith, a researcher with the Nuffield Institute and an expert on the integration of complementary medicine into mainstream medicine, says: 'The financial hammer has come down and health authorities are desperately trying to claw back money. Back in 1991 when the first health reforms to allow doctors to purchase healthcare started to kick in, complementary medicine received a big boost, but it can be difficult for certain patients to get access to NHS-funded treatment now.'

However, Dr Smith is not too despondent. He feels that though funding is tough just now, it will be made easier in the future. Here he is in concurrence with Janet Richardson, who ran a unit in Lewisham in East London, which offered complementary medicine on the NHS to patients referred on by their doctors. Her positive outlook is all the more remarkable considering this unit was recently shut down because of health authority cut backs. 'The point is that now doctors have seen for themselves that complementary medicine works, they want to carry on prescribing it,' she says. 'Doctors have been given much more power by recent legislative changes, and they won't go back. For instance, in our area, a group of them have got together to form a multi-fund to purchase complementary medicine from therapists with NHS funds because they still want their patients to have access to it although the unit is closed.'

More of these sort of schemes will start up in the future and already doctors have found some very inventive ways of getting free complementary medicine treatment for their patients. However, you will need to play detective to a certain extent to find these schemes. Your own doctor may be able to point you in the right direction, even if he doesn't have links with complementary medicine. Otherwise, your local health authority may be able to help.

HOW TO GET TREATMENT FUNDED
BY THE NATIONAL HEALTH SERVICE

1 Ask your doctor. He or she may already have links with complementary medicine.

2 If there are no links, write to your local health authority and find out if there is a unit operating in your area, to which your doctor could refer you.

3 If this proves futile, then you could consider changing doctors. There may be a practice near you which is more open to complementary medicine and you can ask to be put on their list. Your local health authority should be able to help you.

Fund-holding doctors have elected to manage their own budgets. This gives them the flexibility to purchase the services of other health care professionals on behalf of their patients. Many doctors are already convinced of the cost-effectiveness of complementary medicine and may have therapists attached to their practice; some, however, are not, and if unconvinced of its cost-effectiveness are unlikely to be open to the idea.

FUND-HOLDING SCHEMES

Non-fundholding doctors have not opted to manage their own budget but can still apply to the health authority to pay for money to fund complementary therapy for their patients. Such referrals are called ECRs (extra contractual referrals). However, in recent years, lack of funding has made this less likely.

If your doctor refers you to a named therapist, you can be pretty sure that he will have checked out their qualifications, their experience and whether they are insured first. The law is not clear on this, but there is a good case to be made that if any harm should come to you during treatment by a therapist, your doctor will be responsible if he cannot demonstrate that he did all that could be done to ensure that the therapist was qualified. However, it does no harm to check yourself and the details of what you should look for in a therapist are given in the next section.

DOCTORS TRAINED IN COMPLEMENTARY MEDICINE

The easiest way of getting complementary medicine on the National Health Service is if your own doctor or one of his partners is trained in a complementary therapy and offers it as an added service to their patients. The most common therapy in which doctors choose to train is homoeopathy followed by acupuncture.

Having treatment this way can work extremely well. Patients are often delighted by the results and doctors feel they are doing all they can to heal their patients which is why they got into medicine in the first place. But while it is laudable that so many busy doctors have taken the effort to train in their own time in another discipline, it should be remembered that they have rarely trained in anything like the degree that a therapist would have done (many of the courses are done over a few weekends). Although they can offer often excellent, quick relief for certain ailments (and often only claim to do this), for treatment that requires a longer term, holistic approach, there is no substitute for a properly trained therapist.

There are worries within the complementary therapy world and among doctors interested in complementary medicine that there is an element of some doctors trying to get involved too quickly. For instance, there has been a lot of recent debate over the acupuncture point on the wrist P6. P6 is known to be excellent for curing nausea and vomiting. It works so well in fact that it has been suggested that a doctor who knew nothing about acupuncture could easily utilize it. This would, on the surface, appear to be the perfect, simple way of integrating complementary and orthodox medicine, but in theory, it has proven difficult to instigate. It is taking a Western 'quick fix' mentality and applying it to something that can't be quantified that way. As Dr Fiona Bolden, a doctor who practises acupuncture herself, says: 'The reason acupuncture works so well is that the whole basis of it is treating patients as a whole. It is slightly missing the point (no pun intended) to stick in a needle in isolation from the rest of that patient's needs'.

As long as the patient benefits, there is not much need for concern, but there is a worry that some patients who could receive great benefit from a therapy administered by an expert will write off a therapy after failed treatment by an inexperienced practitioner, albeit a medically qualified one.

CHOOSING A COMPLEMENTARY THERAPIST

There are two questions which have to be answered when deciding on a therapist:

- Is he or she qualified in their particular therapy?
- Does he or she instil confidence in you?

The first one is fairly easy. The complementary field is still finding its way when it comes to standardizing levels of training, but now it is reasonably simple to check what sort of training the therapist has had. At the end of this chapter, there are some guidelines to help you.

The question of confidence is a far more nebulous one. But if you want to give yourself the best chance of getting better, you must look for a therapist you can trust and have a rapport with.

Here are some hints from some of the therapists interviewed in this book. They were asked what they whould look out for in a good therapist. They did, however, point out that the best method of finding a good therapist was personal recommendation – there is no substitute for the confidence you will feel knowing that your therapist has already helped someone whose opinion you trust.

- 'Your therapist should be open to orthodox medicine and other therapies. If she gives the impression that her treatment is the only answer, don't go to her.'
- 'No good therapist would expect a patient going through a personal crisis to make drastic changes in their diet or lifestyle.'
- 'A therapist should really listen to what you're saying. If you get any indications that she hasn't been listening to you properly, try someone else.'
- 'A good therapist should be flexible. After a period of treatment, you will change and she should be able to see the changes in you,

and work with them. She should not have a rigid view of what you're about as different priorities will emerge. She should give you the opportunity to change and explore. She mustn't be dogmatic and bossy. You are both working together towards a goal and her language and the way she treats you should reflect that.'

● 'The therapy session should be all about you. After the first session, there's a tendency for patients to feel they have to make small talk. This is fine, but if you don't feel like it, don't bother. You don't have to feel any responsibility towards the therapist. You are paying good money to have your own needs answered, and often this is the only hour in the week when that happens, so relax. You build up a bond after a while and women especially feel that they have to show an interest in their therapist's life because she is showing an interest in theirs! But you are there to focus on you and your health, and a good therapist will always, gently, bring the conversation back to you.'

● 'You should feel comfortable with your therapist, and you should look forward to your session.'

FORMING A 'CONTRACT' WITH YOUR THERAPIST

At the end of your first session, your therapist should know whether she thinks she can help you or not. If she thinks this is possible, you have reached the point of forming a 'contract'. You find out what the treatment will involve and decide if you wish to continue with their treatment. That is your part in the 'bargain'. The therapist has to give you some idea what you are agreeing to, but first find out four things.

● What he or she thinks is wrong with you.
● How he or she intends to treat it.
● Roughly how many sessions he or she thinks will be necessary, and how much each session will cost. The initial session is longer and usually more expensive, subsequent sessions are cheaper.
● Other changes in your lifestyle that might help. (This may not be broached right away. Therapists often concentrate on strengthening your system before they give you such advice which can be difficult to follow when you are feeling low.)

The number of sessions you will need can be problematic. Therapists, especially those trained in Traditional Chinese Medicine, do not have the 'fix-it' mentality that we have in the West. They may well feel that they can offer quick relief, but they don't think that just relieving the main symptom which has brought you to them is enough. They will want to carry on treating you until any underlying weaknesses in your body are rectified and your system is strengthened sufficiently so that you shouldn't get ill again. In the case of long-standing problems this can take months.

However, most patients, quite understandably, get a bit worried at the thought of continuing expensive treatment indefinitely. The way that most experienced therapists deal with this dilemma is to suggest that after six sessions, you will both evaluate the success of the treatment so far and decide if it is worth continuing. (Many patients feel sufficiently better that they are happy to continue treatment for longer than they had originally envisaged.)

Complementary therapy when undertaken privately can prove costly. Those who feel that it is working well for them are usually happy to make sacrifices to continue with their treatment, but in the cases where a patient is deriving benefit but simply can't afford the treatment, some therapists operate a 'sliding scale' of costs depending on the patient's means. They may be willing to lower their charges for you to continue treatment. This is very much up to individual therapists. The prices indicated below are a rough guide and vary greatly depending on where you live and the therapist concerned.

HOW TO FIND A REPUTABLE THERAPIST

Before starting treatment you should find out the following.

● What training your therapist has undergone and whether he or she is affiliated to a recognized regulating body which has its own code of ethics.
● Whether he or she is insured to practise.

As mentioned before, the best method of finding a therapist is through the recommendation of a friend. Besides checking their membership of a reputable professional body, it's worth checking if the therapist is affiliated to the British Complementary Medical Association or Institute for Complementary Medicine, two umbrella organizations for many complementary therapies, with their own code of practice (see page 153).

You can write to one of the organizations listed below to find a local therapist. They will normally respond quickly, but it will speed things up if you enclose a large SAE.

ACUPUNCTURE

There are various organizations which can advise you. A good place to start is the British Acupuncture Council. Their members have to prove their competency to a high standard. Qualifications to look for include BAc, DipAc or LicAc.

Contact:
The British Acupuncture Council
Park House, 206–208 Latimer Road, London W10 6RE
Tel: 0181 964 0222

British Medical Acupuncture Society
Newton House, Newton Lane, Whitley,
Warrington, Cheshire WA4 4JA
Tel: 01925 730 727
(The Society runs acupuncture courses for doctors and dentists and can supply names of those who have completed training.)

Cost of treatment
Acupuncture costs around £40 to £50 for an initial consultation and about £20 to £35 for subsequent sessions.

CLINICAL ECOLOGY

The main society is a combined organization for doctors interested in this field. Your doctor can write to them on your behalf for a referral.

Contact:
The British Society for Allergy, Environmental and Nutritional Medicine
PO Box 28, Totton, Southampton SO40 2ZA
Tel: 01703 812124

Cost of treatment
You may be able to get an NHS referral. Otherwise cost varies wildly for private consultation. Expect to pay around £40 to £60 for a consultation and initial testing may be extra.

HEALING

Many healers aren't members of any organization, but if you can't find one by word of mouth, the National Federation of Spiritual Healers may be able to help. To join, a healer has to have independent evidence of having positively helped at least four people.

Contact:
NFSH
Old Manor Farm Studio, Church Street, Sunbury on Thames,
Middlesex TW16 6RG
Tel: 0891 616080

Cost of treatment
Some healers may work free of charge or ask you to pay only what you can afford.

HERBALISM
Western herbalism
Look for the qualifications MNIMH or FNIMH which denotes membership of the National Institute of Medical Herbalists.

Contact:
The National Institute of Medical Herbalists
56 Longbrook Street, Exeter, EX4 6AH
Tel: 01392 426022
(The Institute can supply you with details of herbalists in your area.)

Cost of treatment

The cost varies between £20 and £35 a session, although the first consultation is usually more expensive than subsequent treatment. The herbs cost extra but are usually inexpensive.

Chinese herbalism

There is no recognized qualification for Chinese herbalists but you can contact the register below.

Contact:

The Register of Chinese Herbal Medicine,
PO Box 400, Wembley, Middlesex, HA9 9NZ
Send a SAE and cheque for £2.50 to receive a list of practitioners.

Cost of treatment

The first consultation is around £30, but following ones are usually quite a bit cheaper.

HOMOEOPATHY

Look for a homoeopath who is registered with the Society of Homoeopaths – they will have the letters RSHom or FSHom – which has stringent joining procedures.

Contact:

The Society of Homoeopaths
2 Artizan Road, Northampton NN1 4HU
Tel: 01604 21400

Medically qualified homoeopaths have the initials MFHom or FFHom after their names.

Contact:

The Faculty of Homoeopathy
2 Powis Place, London WC1N 3HT
Tel: 0171 837 9469

There are five homoeopathic hospitals in Britain: London, Glasgow, Liverpool, Bristol and Tunbridge Wells. You can be referred for NHS treatment to one of these, or you may be able to get a doctor's referral to a local doctor who practises homoeopathy.

Cost of treatment
If you go privately expect to pay £30 to £50 for a first consultation and between £20 and £30 for follow-up appointments.

OSTEOPATHY

Qualified osteopaths have the letters DO (Diploma of Osteopathy) after their name or BSc (Ost). Cranial osteopaths should have the same qualifications but have trained further in cranial osteopathy. Medical doctors who have trained in osteopathy at the London College of Osteopathic Medicine have the letters MLCOM.

Contact:
The Osteopathic Information Service
PO Box 2074, Reading, Berkshire, RG1 4YR
(Write to the Service for a comprehensive register of osteopaths and cranial osteopaths.)

Osteopathy is in a state of flux at the moment as there are four organizations which osteopaths join, all confusingly, with different letters after their name, but these will disappear shortly. The above academic qualification is almost certainly proof enough that a therapist is bona fide but you can double check with the Osteopathic Information Service which only has listings of osteopaths affiliated to the main organizations.

CHIROPRACTIC

Chiropractic is in a similar state of flux. You should look for the qualifications DC or BSc which indicates that the practitioner has undergone training at a recognized college.

Contact:
The British Chiropractic Association
Equity House, 29 Whitley St, Reading, Berkshire RG2 OEG
Tel: 01189 757557
(The Association can put you in touch with a chiropractor in your area.)

The McTimoney Chiropractic Association
21 High St, Eynsham, Oxon OX8 1HE
Tel: 01865 880974

Cost of treatment
You may be able to get osteopathy on the NHS and in the future NHS
access to osteopathy and chiropractic is set to increase. The cost of
going privately is currently around £20 to £40 per session, although you
will probably pay a little more than the therapist's going rate for the
first session.

MIND–BODY THERAPIES
Hypnotherapy
Hypnotherapy training is a very grey area at present. Unless you can get a
recommendation from someone you trust, it is probably advisable to look
for a doctor or dentist who has trained in hypnotherapy.

Contact:
British Society of Medical and Dental Hypnosis
17 Keppel View Road, Kimberworth, Rotherham S612AR
Tel: 01709 554558

Cost of classes
Class rates vary greatly. Therapists' rates vary, too, but expect to pay
around £30 per session.

Yoga
These two organizations can put you in touch with reputable yoga
teachers and remedial yoga therapists.

British Wheel of Yoga
1 Hamilton Place, Boston Road, Sleaford NG34 7ES
Tel: 01529 306851

Yoga for Health Foundation
Ickwell Bury, Ickwell Green, Biggleswade SG18 9EF
Tel: 01767 6277271

Cost of classes
Class rates begin around £4 to £5. Expect to pay around £30 per session.

NUTRITIONAL MEDICINE
The Society for the Promotion of Nutritional Therapy is the leading organization for nutritional therapists.

Contact:
The Society for the Promotion of Nutritional Therapy
PO Box 47, Heathfield, East Sussex TN21 8ZX
Tel: 01825 872921
(Send a SAE and cheque for £1 for a list of members.)

The British Society for Allergy, Environmental and Nutritional Medicine. See page 149 for details.

Cost of treatment
The initial cost of treatment is about £40 for the first session and about £20 to £35 thereafter, although you will have to pay for any supplements prescribed.

IF YOU HAVE A COMPLAINT ABOUT YOUR TREATMENT

The practitioner does not have to give you any guarantee that you will be cured. Indeed, you should avoid one who does. This can be frustrating for patients who don't feel they have benefited from their treatment. If you feel you are being treated unsatisfactorily, first speak to your practitioner who may able to alter the treatment to accommodate your complaints.

If you are still unhappy, complain in writing to the therapist's professional or regulatory body. You can also complain to the umbrella organizations to which the practitioner may belong. The British Complementary Medical Association (Tel: 0116 242 5406) is the most independent. One of its functions is to put you in touch with a qualified therapist but it also has a code of conduct and a disiciplinary procedure for its members to follow. The Institute for Complementary Medicine (Tel: 0171 237 5165) is the other main body and it too claims to take seriously any complaint by the public against one of its associates. Should you have attended the therapist through your doctor's referral, you can use the NHS complaints' procedure to complain.

If you are still not happy and feel that you have a more serious problem or are the victim of negligence, you may want to consider criminal prosecution. You will have to discuss it with a solicitor who works in that area. Action for Victims of Medical Accidents can advise (Tel: 0181 291 2793). But remember, you are unlikely to have a case if you have simply failed to get better. As in all branches of medicine there are no guarantees for a cure. If you can prove on the other hand, that your practitioner did guarantee to heal you, and failed, then you may be able to successfully prosecute them for misleading you.

YOUR PART IN THE THERAPY

Orthodox medicine is a remarkably passive form of medicine. We do what our doctors tell us and if the treatment doesn't work, both doctor and patient tend to blame the drug involved.

Other systems of medicine, notably Chinese, expect the patient to help in their treatment by making lifestyle changes. If you can, try to follow your therapist's advice as it will speed up treatment.

No one is saying this is easy. We do not see food as our medicine, and in the case of, say, chocolate and coffee, we don't see them as our drugs either. But to the therapist, that's exactly what they are.

It is hard for us to believe that foods we enjoy can really do us any harm. To a Chinese physician used to working in the East, it is incredible that when asked to give up chocolate, we in the West continue to eat it. Jill, an acupuncturist tells of the heart-sinking reaction she felt on phoning a patient one evening. This patient had been having acupuncture to help the success of the IVF treatment she was undergoing. That morning she had been into hospital to be implanted with fertilized eggs. 'How are you?' said the acupuncturist. 'Absolutely fine,' said the patient, 'I'm in bed taking it easy, and I've just eaten a huge bowl of strawberries and cream.' This patient had been advised to cut out dairy products and had managed it fairly successfully, but rightly feeling she deserved a treat, had temporarily 'forgotten' her dietary restrictions. 'I couldn't believe it,' said her acupuncturist. 'Obviously, I didn't say anything as I would have only upset her pointlessly, but after working in China, it really brought it home to me how different attitudes are here, in the West.'

With complementary medicine, treatment is a partnership and if you can, work with your therapist by following their advice as far as possible. Be honest, about your inability to give up certain foods or your failure to get to bed early. Part of their job is to help you make these changes and they may be able to give you some worthwhile tips.

Your attitude towards treatment is important, too. Dr Peter Whorwell, the gastroenterologist who has excellent results in his unit treating irritable bowel syndrome with hypnotherapy, asks patients to practise hypnotherapy every day at home between sessions. He can tell if a patient has been cooperating. 'Some people can't be bothered and it shows,' he says. 'They think of hypnosis as like another drug, doled out by their doctor. But ultimately the patient is healing themselves and that takes effort on their part.'

A POSITIVE ATTITUDE

Therapists hope that their patients will have a positive attitude towards their treatment. As Steve, an acupuncturist and homoeopath explains, a negative attitude may be masking underlying problems which ultimately can hinder healing.

'It's important to remember that not every patient wants to be cured. That sounds very harsh – but I sincerely believe that in some cases, where emotional factors are playing a part in the illness then successful treatment depends on the patient having reached the point in their life when they are ready to address these emotional issues. I realized this in my first year as a therapist. A patient came to me with very bad asthma and eczema. This man had done the rounds of every kind of therapist and no one had managed to help him. On our third session, I was trying to take his blood pressure. He was quite a beefy chap and I was having difficulty getting a proper reading from him. Meanwhile, he was becoming increasingly irritated. Eventually, he hissed, 'Look there is the vein right there.' I explained I was taking a reading from his artery, not the vein. But just as I said it, it dawned on me that ever since he'd been coming to see me this man had repeatedly found fault with me. He had come to my clinic expecting me to fail. I decided to have a very frank heart-to-heart talk to him in as sensitive a way as possible get to the root of his negative attitude.

'To cut a long story short, it transpired that this man had been abandoned by his mother at a very young age. In very simple 'psycho-speak', I believe he had real trouble trusting anyone in case they let him down further. He wasn't prepared to trust in the process of getting well. He felt safer hanging onto his illness even though it made him miserable.

'Talking about his mother for the first time in years seemed to do him good and it helped our patient–therapist relationship. We continued treatment and his illnesses improved a bit. But I bumped into him recently at a health show and he is still doing the rounds of therapies looking for an answer, without ever really trusting in the final outcome.

'It is true that those who go into treatment with hopeful expectations, tend to do better than patients who don't expect to get any better. This does not necessarily mean that the patient has to believe in the therapy. But if they give it every chance to succeed, despite their scepticism, they are more likely to do well.' Yoga therapist, Kitty Kennedy thinks this idea of attitude and patient responsibility can be misinterpreted. 'It sounds very much like you're saying to the patient, "It's your fault that you're ill", she says. But of course that isn't the case. It is much more subtle than that. I believe that people reach a point in their lives where they can be helped by the right therapist. If they've reached that point, they will find the help they need, even if it takes time. The search can be part of the healing process. But if they haven't reached that point, they can be treated by the best therapist available without getting any better.

'A good therapist is a guide. Their job is to help the patient unblock anything physical or psychological that blocks the energy flow. This includes mental patterns of thinking that aren't necessarily doing the patient any good. It can feel to the patient that these patterns were put there by the Universe, when in fact they are down to the patient's own experience. Patients come gradually to see that it is their choice whether they stick with these habits of thinking or not.

'But the patients want primarily to get better and so I begin with the physical work. Once the patient starts to feel the energy rebalancing – once they start to experience their own energy flowing smoothly – everything else follows. The body is at ease and that brings vitality. When that happens, if there are any emotional blocks, the patient has the space and strength to deal with them as they surface. The body is very often the patient's doorway into understanding how the body, mind and spirit are all linked.

'But the therapist's job primarily is to approach and relieve the immediate physical stress which the patient is suffering. Anything else that follows is a continuing process and the patient does the work. The therapist simply offers the support and guidance which makes that work possible.'

Dr Brenda Davies, psychiatrist and healer believes that:

'Illness is often a sign that the methods we have used to cope in the past aren't working any more. We get spiritual "messages", then emotional "messages" that there is something demanding our attention, and if we ignore them, we finally get physical "messages". Orthodox medicine is very useful for treating physical symptoms but the danger is that only the physical messages are dealt with and the emotional and spiritual ones remain unaddressed. However, there are always ways of treating the physical problems, so that the emotional and spiritual ones are healed, too.'

references

ILLNESSES

Anxiety
1. Abbey, 1982. J Orthomol Psychiat. 11: 243–259.
2. Hoes et al, 1981. J Orthomol Psychiat. 10 (1): 7–15.
3. Simington and Laing, 1993. Clin Nursing Research. 2 (4), 438–450.

Arthritis
Osteoarthritis
1. Gaw et al, 1975. New Eng J Med. 293 (8), 375–378.
2. Lewith and Machin, 1983. Acup Electro Therap Res. 6 (4), 277–284.
3. Milligan et al, 1981. Fifteenth International Congress of Rheumatology, Paris.
4. Varma et al, 1988. Br Homoeopathic J. 77 (1), 27–29.
5. Machtey and Ouaknine, 1978. J Ann Geriat Soc. 26, 328.
6. Gibson et al, 1980. Practitioner. 234, 955–960.
7. Bingham et al, 1975. J Appl Nutr. 27, 45–50.
Rheumatoid Arthritis
1. Lewith, 1984. Roy Coll Gen Pract. 34, 275–278.
2. Man and Barager, 1974. J Rheum. 1 (1), 126–129.
3. Gibson et al, 1978. Br Clin J Pharmacol. 6, 391-395.
4. Gibson et al, 1980.

Practitioner 234, 955 60.
5. Kjeldsen-Kragh et al, 1991. Lancet. 338, 899–902.
6. Roberts, 1984. Br J Dermatol. 110, 735–736.
7. Johansson et al, 1986. Human Nutr: Coin Nutr. 40C, 57–67.
8. Clemmenson et al, 1980. Br J Dermatol. 103, 411–415.

Asthma
1. Nagarathna and Nagendra, 1985. Br Med J. 291, 172–174.
2. Ewer and Stewart, 1986. Br Med J. 293 (6555), 1129–1132.
3. Simon, 1982. Res Inst Scripps Clin Scient Rep. 39, 57–58. Crocket, 1957. Acta Allergologica. XI: 261–268. Schwartz and Weiss, 1990. Am J Epidemiol. 132 (1), 67–76.
4. Burney, 1989. Thorax. 44 (1), 36–41.
5. Wraith, 1987. Food allergy and intolerance. Balliere Tindall, London.
6. Wraith, 1987. Food allergy and intolerance. Balliere Tindall, London.
7. Kleifnen et al, 1991. Br Med J. 302, 316–323.
8. Reilly et al, 1986. Lancet. 2, 881–886.

Back Pain
1. Meade et al, 1990. Br Med J. 300, 1431–1437.
2. Lewith and Turner, 1982. Practitioner. 226, 1614–1618.
3, Mendelson, 1983. Am J Med. 74, 49–55.
4. Weintraub et al, 1975. Clin Pharmacol Therap. 17, 248.
5. Junnila, 1982. Am J Acupuncture. 10, 259–262.

Bowel Disorders
1. Riordan et al, 1993. Lancet. 342, 1131–1134.
2. McEwen, 1987. Clin Ecol. 5 (2), 47–51.
3. Alun-Jones et al,1982. Lancet. 2, 1115–1117.
4. Whorwell et al, 1984. Lancet. 2, 1232–1234.
5. Ritter et al, 1993. Comp Therap Med. 1 (4), 189–193.

Cancer
1. Filshie, 1990. Acupuncture in Medicine. 8 (2), 38–40.
2. Dundee, 1988. Acupuncture in Medicine. 1, 22–24.
3. Price et al, 1991. Compl Med Res. 5, 93–94.
4. Speigel et al, 1989. Lancet. 2, 888–891.
5. Fawzey et al, 1990. Arch Gen Psych. 47, 720–735.

Candidiasis
1. Dismukes et al, 1990. New Eng J Med. 323 (25), 1717–1723.

Chronic Fatigue Syndrome
1. Behan et al, 1990. Acta Neurol Scand. 82, 209–216.
2. Cox et al, 1991. Lancet. 337, 757–760.
3. Awdry, 1996. Int J Alt Comp Med. 14, 12-160.

Depression
1. Werbach and Murray, 1994.
2. Schubert and Halama, 1993. Geriatr Forsch. 3, 45-53.
3. Carney, 1982. Br J Psychiat. 141, 271–272. Coppen, 1986. J Effective Disord. 10, 9–13.
4. Adams, 1974. Lancet. 2, 516–517
5. Milner, 1963. Br J Psychiat. 109, 294–299.
6. Ossofsky, 1976. Compre Psychiat. 17, 335.
7. Richelson, 1982. J Clin Psychiat. 43, 4.
8. Hann, 1986. Int J Neurosci. 29 (1–2), 79–92.
9. Guangzhi et al, 1992. Journal of Traditional Chinese Medicine. 12 (2) 91–4.

Hay fever
1. Reilly et al, 1986. Lancet. 2, 881–886.
2. Clemetson, 1980. J Nutr. 110 (4) 662—668.
3. Brown and Ruskin, 1949. Ann Allergy. 7, 65–70.
4. Kamimura, 1972. J Vitaminol. 18 (4), 204–209.
5. Amella, 1985. Planta Medica. 51, 16–20.
6. Mittman, 1990. Planta Medica. 56, 44-47.

Hormonal And Fertility
Problems
PMS
1. Brush and Perry, 1985.
Lancet. 1, 1339.
2. Williams et al, 1985. J Int
Med Res. 13, 174–179.
3. Barr, 1984. Practitioner. 228,
425–427.
4. London et al, 1984. J Am
Coll Nutr. 3 (4) 351–356.
5. Nicholas, 1973. First
International Symposium on
Magnesium Deficiency in
Human Pathology, 261–263.
6. Puolakka et al, 1985. J
Reprod Med. 39 (3), 149–153.
7. Horrobin, 1983. J Reprod
Med. 28 (7), 465–468.
8. Weiss, 1988. Herbal
Medicine. Beaconsfield
Publishers, Beaconsfield.
9. Heckel, 1953. Am J Obstet
Gynecol. 66, 1297.
10. Miller, 1974. J Med Assoc
Alla. 44, 57.
11. Rossignol, 1985. Am J
Public Health. 75 (11),
1335–1337.
12. Goei et al, 1982. J Applied
Nutr. 34 (1), 4–11.
13. Ferrannini, 1982. J Cloin
Endocrinol Metab. 54, 455.
14. Goei et al, 1982. J Applied
Nutr. 34 (1), 4–11.
Menopause
1. Bradley, 1992. British Herbal
Compendium Col 1 13. British
Herbal Medical Association.

Hyperactivity
1. Egger et al, 1992. Lancet.
339, 1150–1153.
2. Lewith et al, 1992. The
Complete Guide to food allergy
and food intolerance, 65–75.
Green Print, London.

Migraine
1. Egger et al, 1983. Lancet. 2,
865.
2. Monro et al, 1984. Lancet. 2,
719–721.
3. Hyman et al, 1989. Nursing
Res. 38 (4), 216–220.
4. Sorbi et al, 1989. Headache.
29 (2), 111–121.
5. Olness et al, 1987. Pediatrics.
79 (4), 593–597.
6. Parker et al, 1978. Austral.
NZ Med J. 8 (6), 589–593.
Vincent, 1990. J Psychosom Res.
34, 533–561.
7. Brigo and Serpellion, 1991.
Berlin J REs Homoeop. 1, 2.

Skin disorders
Acne
1. Juhlin and Micheaelsson,
1983. Acta Derm Veneraol. 63:
538–540
2. Basset et al, 1990. Med J
Australia. 153 (8) 455–458
3. Michaelsson and Edquist,
1984. Acta Derm Venerol 64:
9–14
4. Michaelsson et al, 1977. Br J
Dermatol. 96: 283–286
Eczema
1. Wright and Burton, 1982.
Lancet. 1120–1122. Wright,
1985. Acta Derm Venereal
(Stockholm) Suppl. 114,
143–145.

2. Allison, 1945. South Med J. 38, 235–241.
3. Sheehan et al, 1992 Lancet. 340, 13–17.

Psoriasis
1. Proctor et al, 1979. Arch Dermatol. 115: 945–949.
2. Haddox et al, 1979. Cancer Research. 39: 4940–4948. Kuwano and Yamauchi, 1960. Chem Pharm Bull. 8: 491–496.
3. Rao and Field, 1984. Biochem Soc Trans. 12: 177–180.
4. Lithell et al, 1983. Acta Derm Vener. 63: 397–403.
5. Bazex et al, 1976. Ann Derm Symp. 103: 648.
6. Bittiner et al, 1988. Lancet. 378–380. Ziboh et al, 1986. Arch Dermatol. 122: 1277–1282. Maurice et al, 1987.Br J Dermatol. 117: 599–606.
7. Weber and Galle, 1983.Med Welt. 34: 108–111.

PROBLEMS
Insomnia
1. Leatherwood et al, 1982. Pharmacol. Biochem Behav. 17 (1), 65–71.
2. Stone, 1980. Electoencephalogr Clin Neurophysiol. 48 (6), 706–709.
3. Shirlow and Mathers, 1985. Int J Epidemiol. 14 (2), 239–248.
4. Hartmann, 1985. Speaking at a symposium sponsored by the AMA, quoted in Clin Psychiat News, March 1985.

Giving Up Smoking
1. Schwartz, 1988. Am J Acupuncture. 16, 135–142.
2. Lewith and Vincent, 1995. Pain Forum. 4 (1) 29–39.
3. Orne, 1977. Health consequences, cessation activities, and social action. Vol 2. 49. DHEW Publication No. (NIH) 1413–1477.
4. Ryde, 1985. Practitioner. 229, 29–31.
5. Spiegel, 1970. Arch Environ Hlth. 20, 736.
6. Pederson, 1979. Int J Clin Exp Hypn. 27, 14.
7. Kline, 1970. Int J Clin Exp Hypn. 18, 270.

THERAPIES
Homoeopathy
1. Del Giudice et al, 1982. Physics Letters. 90A, 104.

Herbal Medicine
1. Balandrin et al, 1985. Science. 228, 1154–1160.

Nutritional Medicine
1. Reynolds and Natta, 1985. Am J Clin Nutr. 41, 684–688.
2. Britton et al, 1994. Lancet. 344, 357–362.
3. Stich et al, 1991. Am J Clin Nutr. 53 (1 Suppl), 298–304.
4. Butterworth et al, 1982. Am J Clin Nutr. 35 (1), 73–82.
5. Facchinetti et al, 1991. Obstet Gynecol. 78 (2), 177–181.
6. Nicholas, 1973. First International Symposium on

Magnesium Deficiency in Human Pathology. 261–263. Springer Verlag, Paris.
7. Mason, 1993 Comp Ther Med. 1, 19–23.
8. Riemersma et al, 1991. Lancet. 337, 1–5.

Healing
1. Miller, 1977. Methods of detecting and measuring healing energies. In: Future Science, published by Anchor Doubleday.
2. Patrovsky, 1983. Proceedings of the 5th International Conference on Psychotronic Research. Bratislava, 88–95.
3. Kreiger, 1976. Psychoenergetic systems. 1, 121–129.
4. Wirth, 1990. Research in parapsychology. 47–52.

Clinical Ecology
1. Darlington et al, 1986. Lancet. 1, 236–238.
2. Hunt et al, 1983. In: Second Food Allergy Workshop, 69–72. Medicine Publishing Foundation, Oxford.

Mind–Body Therapies
1. Tinterow, 1987. Kansas Medicine. 6, 190–192.
2. Kabat-Zinn, 1990. Full catastrophe living: using the wisdom of your body and mind to face stress, pain and illness. Delaware Press, New York.
3. Benson et al, 1977. Am Scient. 65, 441–445.
4. Morrison, 1988. Chronic asthma and improvement with relaxation induced by hypnotherapy. JRSM
5. Nagarathna and Nagendra, 1985. BMJ. 291, 172.

index